Sc[illegible]f Taoist Sorcery

To: Xue "Jon"
Best Wishes,
Tony

Contents

~<^><^><^><^><^><^><^><^><^><^><^><^><^><^>~

Introduction

There are certain practitioners that deviate from the original teaching. These are the ones that follow the "Tao of the Left", "Left Handed Paths" or "Side Doors" teachings. They practice sorcery that is extremely fierce. Some of them have great spiritual powers. They can cause the victim to become insane and eventually die a horrible death!

Taoist sorcery comes in many different forms it may be elements such as air, earth, wind and fire combined. They may even use spirits of the deceased to do their bidding, words and sounds (mantra) formulated into certain vibrations to effect a physical change in others, the earth's meridian, astrological constellations, natural energies, guardians, spirits and beings that inhabits the mountain, forest, or even a lake. Taoist Sorcery in a white or black magic form depends on the motivation of the practitioners. It is usually used to fulfill some wish quickly that is impossible to accomplish by normal means.

Christian's, and other religious people think magic is often used as a pejorative term for Pagan rituals, with the implication that they involve sinful, blasphemous or idolatrous practices. Among occultists, magic is a fairly neutral term which has some varied connotations, such as white magic and black magic.

For decades I had researched and found that black magic and sorcery practiced throughout the world share similar rituals, even though they are practiced in different part of the continents. I believe it is from the same sources that had revealed to them regardless of creed, languages and ethnic group.

Some use the voodoo doll sorcery share a similar ritual. An effigy made of straw or other materials are fashion as a representation of the victim, hair, nails or any belongings of the victim are also attached to the doll and most significantly a soul invocation mantra is recited to summon the intended victim soul to be attached to the doll. Needles or pins are then stuck to the doll to inflict harm on the victim. Sorcerer with strong psychic power or spiritual powers can cast this spell and even kill an intended victim living in another part of the continent!

In South East Asia sorcery is rampant. There are numerous types of sorcery practiced, especially love spell or infatuation spell, sorcery to ruin a rival business, sorcery to cause death, insanity, separation, and even to cause a victim impotent!

In Indonesia a renowned type of poison called “Santau” is feared by the community there. Any victims that happen to consume such poison suffer an impending death within three months or even a shorter life-span depending on the toxicity of the poison. This type of poison is most lethal as it is odorless and colorless, it can just blend and dissolve into any food or drinks without causing any suspicion when the intended victim consumed it. The victim internal organs are gradually damaged by the poison as it also contains arsenic, victims tend to cough profusely. The reason is because one of the key ingredient comprise of small particles of shaven bamboo shoots that can cause irritation to the throat.

Can you imagine these small particles get lodged on the throat it would cause infection to the esophagus. The victims shall have several symptoms such as coughing and expelling phlegm together with blood, gradually losing weight, indigestion and insomnia. If left untreated the condition shall worsen and caused death.

The fascinating world of Taoist sorcery is a complex one and it is my hope that I will have shed some light on the often misunderstood mystery of Taoist sorcery.

Plants and sorcery

The fact that plants, in common 'with man and the lower animals, possess the phenomena of life and death, naturally suggested in primitive times, the notion of their having a similar kind of existence In both cases there is a gradual development which is only reached by certain progressive stages of growth, a circumstance which was not without its practical lessons to the early naturalist. This similarity, too, was held all the more striking when it was observed how the life of plants, like that of the higher organisms, was subject to disease, accident, and other hostile influences, and so liable at any moment to be cut off by an untimely end. On this account a personality was ascribed to the products of the vegetable kingdom, survivals of which are still of frequent occurrence at the present day. It was partly this conception which invested trees with that mystic or sacred character whereby they were regarded with a superstitious fear which found expression in sundry acts of sacrifice and worship.

There is reason to believe that " the doctrine of the spirits of plants lay deep in the intellectual history of South-east Asia, but was in great measure superseded under Buddhist influence. The Buddhist books show that in the early days of their religion it was matter of controversy whether trees had souls, and therefore whether they might lawfully be injured. Orthodox Buddhism decided against the tree souls, and consequently against the scruple to harm them, declaring trees to have no mind nor sentient principle, though admitting that certain dewas or spirits do reside in the body of trees, and speak from within them." Anyhow, the notion of its being wrong to injure or mutilate a tree for fear of putting it to unnecessary pain was a widespread belief. Thus, the Ojibways imagined that trees had souls, and seldom cut them down, thinking that if they did so they would hear ' the wailing of the trees when they suffered in this way."

In Sumatra certain trees have special honors paid to them as being the embodiment of the spirits of the woods, and the Fijians believe that if an animal or a plant die, its soul immediately goes to Bolotoo. The Dayaks of Borneo assert that rice has a living principle or spirit, Taoist and Shinto philosophy regarding herbs and plants are that, the "key" is to remain in harmony. With both the environment and the relationship between both the animal or person being treated with the herb, plant or combination of more than one.

It is unfortunate that the terminology of the English language has become skewed when it comes to the word 'sorcerer or sorcery'.

True it is an occult or mystic term, but so does the candle burning and magical transformation of wine into blood, eaten the flesh of a being? Taoist sorcery is merely keeping the human or animal in a state of perfect health by the influence of certain foods, herbs, exercise, and the invocation of sounds (examples of these are 'hua' hum') these sounds are beneficial and will actually realign DNA on a cellular level. The many thousands of years that Taoist masters have known this and only now in the last few years modern science has born this fact out. Words can and do have meaning and power!

Every thought you let cross your mind can be exerted into the physical world. The Buddhist "right thought, right action" is an excellent maxim to adhere to and is easily remembered. Getting back to the sounds, the ancient masters knew that when certain syllables were combined health would be influenced. In Indian yoga the mantra "AUM" is often used. It resonates from the base of the skull to the crown. It serves to enhance the thought process and also again, the DNA is responsive in a positive way.

What Taoist sorcery did (as well as some Buddhist sects) is combine these single syllable sounds into chants, songs, phrases, and words. Common people witnessing the Taoist masters healing people with just a prayer, or speaking words to the ill. Thought (due to ignorance) that it was some 'magical' power coming from the Taoist master and as time went on like all things bits and pieces of information would be added to the legends and thus the secret compounded by time and the uninformed became 'sorcery'. The miraculous powers were much further enhanced by the vast knowledge of herbs and treatment methods. More so by the three big internal martial arts; Tai Ch'i Chuan, Hsing I Chuan, and Bau Gua. Many off shoot martial arts from these has spread around Asia.

The practice of these internal martial arts alone will increase the human body's energy, immunity, and life force or vital force (ch'i, ki, qi, prana, huna, or ka) . The average male will dissipate the vital force they are born with and run out by age 30-40. This is why the age is accelerated vs. not having sex and not being able to replace the vital force used or expended. If the vital force is kept in check the body will remain in good harmony. However, if more of the vital force is expended, than taken in aging and a multitude of health conditions will occur-none of which are good.

In Europe this vital force was also called "la" or spirit. Men and animals have their "la" or spirit (vital energy). The Iroquois acknowledge the existence of spirits in trees and plants, and say that the spirit of beans, and the spirit of squash are supposed to have the forms of three beautiful maidens. According to a tradition current among the Miamis, one year when there was an unusual abundance of corn, the spirit of the corn was very angry because the children had thrown corncobs at each other in play, pretending to have suffered serious bodily injury in consequence of their sport. Similarly, when the wind blows the long grass or waving corn, the German peasant will say, " the Grass- wolf," or " the Corn- wolf " is abroad. According to some places " the last sheaf of rye is left as a shelter to the Roggen-wolf or Eye-wolf during the winter's cold, and in many a summer or autumn festive rite that being is represented by a rustic, who assumes a wolf-like appearance.

The corn-wolf spirit was, however, often symbolized under a human form." Indeed, under a variety of forms this animistic conception is found among the lower races, and in certain cases explains the strong prejudice to certain herbs as articles of food. The Society Islanders ascribed a " varua " or surviving soul to plants, and the Negroes of Congo adored a sacred tree called "Mirrone," one being generally planted near the house, as if it were the tutelar god of the dwelling. It is customary, also, to place calabashes of palm wine at the feet of these trees, in case they should be thirsty. In modem folklore there are many curious survivals of this tree-soul doctrine. In Westphalia, the peasantry announce formally to the nearest oak any death that may have occurred in the family, and occasionally this formula is employed " "The master is dead, the master is dead." Even in past years, writes Sir John Lubbock, an oak copse at Loch Saint, in the Isle of Skye, was held so sacred that no person would venture to cut the smallest branch from it. The Wallachians " have a superstition that every flower has a soul, and that the waterlily is the sinless and scentless flower of the lake, which blossoms at the gates of Paradise to judge the rest, and that she will inquire strictly what they have done with their odors." It is noteworthy, also, that the Indian belief which describes the holes in trees as doors through which the special spirits of those trees pass, reappears in the German superstition that the holes in the oak are the pathways for elves ; and that various diseases may be cured by contact with these holes. Hence some trees are regarded with special veneration " particularly the lime and pine" and persons of a superstitious turn of mind "may often be seen carrying sickly children to a forest for the purpose of dragging them through such holes."

How to prepare Chinese herbs

There are more than a thousand varieties of Chinese medicinal herbs, most of which are gathered by specially trained persons in the great province of Sze Chuan, in Western China. These herbs consist of leaves, bark, berries, and roots, all of which must be cleaned and steamed in order to sterilize them. The roots, moreover, are given a special scrub and then steamed for twenty-four hours. After having been steamed, the herbs are either put into the sun to dry; "or in case the weather is rainy, are dried under shelter in specially constructed ovens.

As a rule, however, the herbs are not put through these processes in the province in which they are gathered, but are shipped immediately to Hong Kong to exporting firms having special facilities for cleaning, cutting, steaming and drying herbs on a large scale, as well as for sanitary packing and for shipping. While the processes to which the herbs are subjected in preparing them for market serve both to remove all foreign matter and to thoroughly sterilize them, they do not, however, rob them of their healing properties or of their delicate fragrance.

When a well-sealed box of these carefully prepared herbs is received in the United States and opened, the room is filled with an aroma comparable only to that of the forests in May. There is one conspicuous difference between Chinese and Occidental herbs. The latter are generally sold in small packages and are ground almost to a powder, while the Chinese herbs from which one cup of tea is made are in large pieces, each leaf, berry, or piece of bark or root being distinct from the others. In fact, a package of Chinese herbs, in- stead of containing two or three teaspoonfuls of powdered herbs, contains about three cupfuls of herbs of approximately twenty varieties, each in its natural color and form. Again, most Occidental herbs are merely steeped before drinking, but in order to make a cup of tea from a package of Chinese herbs, one must add four cups of water and boil them for half an hour, after which they are strained before drinking.

If we cut, grind or boil it, any herb can be eaten without the slightest harm to the human system. When these herbs are compounded by a specialist who has an extensive knowledge of their properties, they work wonders in the regeneration of the body.

No creature can live without vegetation. Because of lack of vegetation on the great deserts, there is no animal life. Vegetation that is mild in taste is used for man's daily food. Some vegetation of sour or bitter taste possesses curative power and is valuable as a corrective. Hundreds of varieties of herbs are used as foods. Anyone who doubts this statement can make the test by ordering Chinese dishes at any good Chinese restaurant. The wholesome and delicious Chinese Herb dishes are unequaled in bodybuilding value by any other foods.

I have heard many persons say: "I have no confidence in herbs." These people do not stop to think that most of their daily food is of vegetable origin, and that even fish, meat, milk, butter, and sugar come under this head. If there were no vegetation, neither cattle nor fish could subsist. It would seem as if those people who do not believe in herbs do not believe in the wisdom of God, who gives us vegetation so freely. Furthermore, how can they believe that their strength and vitality can be maintained by eating three meals a day? Besides our common food and the remedial herbs, the building material and furniture of our homes and the beautiful flowers in our gardens all belong to the vegetation element. Without vegetation, there would be no fuel; neither could minerals be welded into instruments.

The colors of flowers attract the human sense of sight. They correspond to the colors of the human organs. Green, besides being the most prevalent and most restful color, has the greatest attraction .for the human eye. Green is the vegetation color. The liver belongs to the vegetation of the body. Therefore, the liver is also attracted by the color green. The Chinese believe that the colors in the eyes represent the colors of the internal organs. For instance, the color of the iris represents the color of the liver; the white of the eye represents the light color of the lungs; and the dark pupil represents the color and strength of the kidneys. Therefore, various colors attract not only the human eye, but also the senses of the internal organs.

Why do children like sweets ? Because the stomach and the spleen are yellow, thus resembling the color of the earth element. The taste of the earth is sweet; therefore, the stomach and the spleen naturally develop earlier and with greater rapidity than any of the other organs. Children like sweet things almost immediately after birth. The liver belongs to the vegetation element. The taste of vegetation is sour.

When a person craves sour food, his liver has need of them. The kidneys and the bladder belong to the water element. The taste of urine and of water is salty. When a person craves salt ,the kidneys and the bladder are in need of it. Just as the organs crave various food elements, even so are they attracted by the different colors. If any organ in the human body fails to function properly, Nature's herbal remedies are required to revitalize it.

The difference between drugs and herbs

Naturally ,when we look at the words "drug" and "herb," we think of them as being related. Each consists of four letters. There, how- ever, the resemblance ends. A herb is an organic substance of vegetable origin. It has life and it supplies nourishment for the building up and strengthening of the body.

It also eliminates poisons from the human system. A herb is a food, which, if eaten correctly, eradicates and prevents many ailments. A herb belongs to the vegetation element and can be grown in many different localities. It has no habit-forming or other bad effects.

A drug is usually of mineral origin and is an inorganic substance. Sometimes, however, a drug is derived from vegetables or herbs, but only through a chemical process. It has no life and has a deadening or killing effect. A drug is frequently a poison which at times is used to destroy other poisons. Therefore, the after effects are often harmful.

Extracts of various Chinese herbal remedies have been subjected to chemical processes in order to precipitate their elements. However, many kinds of herbs and roots show nothing in the test tube; consequently, the chemists cannot determine their uses. For example a chemist is never able to discover the elements in the Ginseng Root which is a wonderful remedy in building up the air circulation in the body. For the past 5,000 years, the Chinese have used ginseng root to strengthen the air circulation and have combined it with other herbal remedies to improve the blood circulation.

Articles written by chemists or pharmacists frequently appear in the newspapers ridiculing the Chinese as being superstitious in believing that ginseng has great medicinal value. Because these writers cannot see the curling of the smoke, they say there is no fire.

In this twenty-first century, human suffering may be classified under three groups,;

(1) Neuritis, headaches, nerve pains in the back of the neck or in the head, or pain in the shoulder blades. These pains are generally due to either inflammation of the blood stream or to the improper functioning of the kidneys and the bladder. Generally, these conditions are not manifest in either blood tests or urine tests. In consequence, patients are told that their kidneys and bladders are in good condition.

(2) The blood around the valves of the heart becomes poisoned, heated by the fire element, and congested. Pains run through the chest, the nerves, the arms and the shoulder blades.

(3) The improper functioning of the liver or of the gall bladder. The pain runs along the right side through the back and more or less through the stomach. Persons suffering from the aforesaid ailments, having failed to secure relief, are generally advised to have even their good teeth extracted, their tonsils removed (even though they may be small in size),the gall bladder drained, the appendix removed, and one kidney taken out. Yet, after all this, they still suffer. The basic causes are to be found in the blood stream.

The result of having teeth extracted is faulty mastication, faulty digestion and broken health. How many persons are free from suffering after the gall bladder has either been drained or taken out? How many young people who have their appendices removed become subject to either nervous attacks or to epileptic fits? How many little folks who have had their tonsils removed have either died or had their eyes sunken in? Lacking a fundamental knowledge of their ailments, people are led by so-called medical advisers just as the blind lead the blind. Is this to be regarded as advance in twentieth century science ?

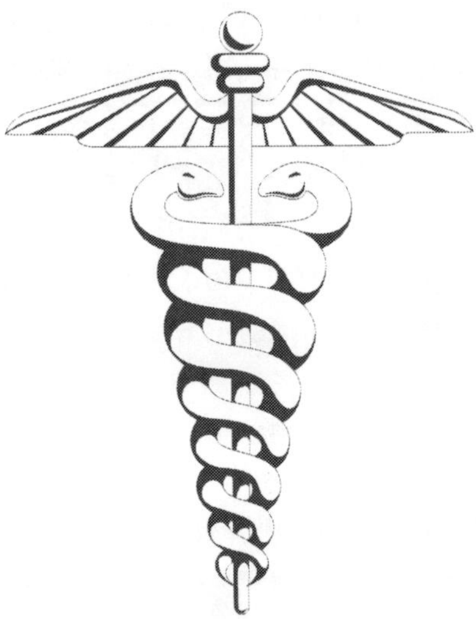

Ginseng is used to increase the circulation

As far back as the beginning of Chinese civilization, the people of China had learned through their herbalists that in the bodies of all living creatures there are two circulations; i.e.,the circulation of the blood and that of the breath. In the ancient literature on herbs we find the statement, "Man's blood is his glory; his breath is his protection".

If the circulation of either of these is impeded, the five viscera do not function normally and the system becomes poisoned. In the many Chinese methods of treatment, the circulation of the breath is deemed of more importance than that of the blood, because if the breath circulation is impeded, the blood cannot follow, just as in a water pipe, unless the air goes through first the water cannot make its way.

In Occidental schools of medicine, the scientists frequently say that such and such a person is anemic or lacks blood. Moreover, we often hear people say, "I am short-winded and cannot get my breath." However, the medical men never claim that the short-winded person lacks breath or air. On the other hand, when a person is anemic, blood-transfusion is commonly resorted to; while sometimes iron is injected to build up the blood or electrolytes applied to the body to accelerate the circulation of the blood. Again, the sufferer may be advised to drink alcoholic liquors, or even the fresh warm blood of a calf, freshly sauntered.

On the other hand, we never hear of people who are short of

breath being taken to a service station to have air pumped into their bodies. In fact, nothing is done to increase the air supply in the system. If the Chinese theories are correct, Occidental Medical Science, which omits the study of the breath or air circulation, is only 50% efficient, even granting that its methods of building up the blood are successful.

While expensive deer antler is used as a blood restorer in China, herbs compounded for this purpose have proven more successful and are commonly used.

In the Chinese herb treatment various kinds of ginseng roots are used to strengthen the air circulation and restore the power to the breath. In order that the blood may not become inflamed, ginseng of the more common varieties is generally compounded with different kinds of herbs to produce blood and air in people who are run-down and weak. In the Occident, people who are weak and sick are often given iron tonics or injections of iron, which cause headache and pain in the nerves of the neck and temples, together with afternoon fever, red lips, and hot cheeks.

The Chinese know positively that ginseng is a Tonic and restorative. The highest-priced North China Ginseng costs $1000. per ounce!

This makes but one cup of Ginseng Tonic. Millions of dollars worth of intensive studies and carrying on numerous experiments in order to determine scientifically the exact effects of certain Chinese Herbs upon the human system.

Ma Huang is another good herb, the curative powers of this

plant should be investigated further. The manner in which Ma Huang is used by the Chinese in Herbal Compounds is quite different from the ways that the Americans use it (or abuse it making ephedrine and then methamphetamine) in combination with other things. The Chinese method is not harmful.

Chaulmoogra oil, Digitalis, Ephedrine, Mercury, Salvarsan plus many other drugs and herbal combinations have been used in China for thousands of years. However, during the past few centuries, the use of Mercury and Salvarsan has been gradually abandoned, as the Chinese have discovered that these drugs contain too much poison for the human system to cope with.

The Chinese have therefore resorted more and more to herbs, which, while having great healing power, leave none of the bad after effects common to drugs. Digitalis, an extract of Foxglove Root, is beneficial to the heart. Ephedrine is an extract from the Chinese herb "Ma Huang."

Chaulmoogra Oil for leprosy, so recently acclaimed by the Western World, was known to the Chinese long before any foreigner ever visited China. The Chinese Encyclopedia of Herbal Science, which was published by the Chinese Govern-
A branch from the Cltaulmoogra tree, showing seeds from which it Is extracted. Chaulmoogra Oil, is but one illustration of the fact the Chinese possessed knowledge of medicinal remedies far in advance of western science and that many of the so-called "new discoveries" in West are ‘old news’.

The compass an Chinese herbal remedies

The compass was invented by the Chinese many thousands of years ago; yet not only do the world's aviators use this Chinese invention to guide them, but it is also used by ships, warships, engineering works, and even in getting direction for long range guns. All nations, great and small, use this invention to help them find their way in the world.

Now that the world is gradually awakening to the value of Chinese herbs, the young Chinese students in the Medical Colleges are frequently asked by the doctors under whom they study what one or another kind of herb is used for. While these medical men are deeply interested in the scraps of information thus gleaned, they do not realize that these Chinese students are not herbalists and that they know only a little of but a very few kinds of the herbs that are used by the Chinese to relieve human suffering.

Moreover, these few kinds of herbs in the hands of Occidental doctors are comparable to what a few selections from English Literature would be to a Chinese who had just learned his A B C's. Even though these medical men might learn the uses of hundreds of kinds of Chinese herbs, yet, because of their lack of fundamental and experimental knowledge of herb treatment, they would soon forget what they had learned, and the five thousand formulas that have been worked out by ancient Chinese Herbalists would be valueless to them.

While the use of the Chinese invention, the compass, has never been attacked and prohibited because of jealousy, the practice of Chinese herbs is continually under fire, for the reason that practitioners in other schools of healing realize that the marvelous success of the herb treatments has shorn them of much of their business.

These attacks, but has gained the applause, gratitude and friendship of thousands of Americans. Just as the compass is so efficient that it cannot be either improved upon or replaced by something modern, neither can a substitute be found for the ancient Chinese herbal remedies nor their formulas changed and improved. May it not be in the not far distant future that the medical men of the world will discover that Chinese herbs and ancient Chinese methods of healing surpass the newer medical discoveries just as the ordinary compass "beats all new instruments" as a guide to direction?

The human and Chinese musical tones

It is a matter of common information that the ancient Chinese based their knowledge of herbal remedies upon the relationship between the five principal internal organs of the human body and the five natural elements; i.e., the Mineral, Vegetation, Water, Fire and Earth elements.

However, very few people know that the ancient Chinese went so far as to base the five principal musical tones (1, Kok; 2, Ching; 3, Kong; 4, Sheng; 5, Yii) upon the five principal elements in connection with the internal organs of the human system.

The first one, Kok, is identified with the vegetation element and is related to the liver;

The second, Ching, with the fire element (the heart) ;

The third, Kong, with the earth element (the stomach and the spleen) ;

The fourth, Sheng, with the mineral element (the lungs); and

The fifth, Yii, with the water element (the kidneys).

If a Chinese musician plays without knowing how the five principal musical tones were derived, he lacks ability to appeal to the five principal organs of the human system. Likewise, the Chinese Herbalist who lacks a fundamental knowledge of the five principal elements and their relation to the five principal human organs is incapable of detecting the ailments of those sufferers who are in such pain that they cannot talk coherently but only groan and murmur.

Five colors represent the five elements in nature

1. Red represents the fire element.
2. Yellow represents the earth element.
3. Black (dark) represents the water element.
4. White represents the mineral element.
5. Greenish brown represents the vegetation element.

Not only does each of these colors represent an element in nature but it also represents one of the five divisions of the human race. Therefore, in each human race, one or more of these five colors is present.

For example: Some individuals of the Caucasian race are very white; others are a darkish brown (liver color), while others are a greenish white, a yellowish white, or a reddish white. In each person, there is a combination of one dominant color with others of these five colors.

A red, inflamed face signifies that the blood is overheated, there being too much of the fire element. This condition causes nervousness, high blood pressure, headache, dizziness and heart trouble. Persons with a liver-colored or with a yellowish-green complexion are victims of ailments of the gall bladder and spleen.

In addition to the fact that the majority of internal disorders are made manifest by the color of the skin, it is also true that the color of the human tongue reveals the condition of the internal organs. For thousands of years, Chinese Herbalists have studied the colors of the tongue, because it is possible in many cases to discover with certainty the diseased conditions of the internal organs by simply looking at the tongue.

The key to the method of "tongue-reading" is as follows : The color of the tip of the tongue represents the heart; of the center, the stomach and spleen; of the edges, the liver and gall; and of the under-side of the tongue, the kidneys. A brownish color signifies an over-heated system. Not infrequently do tongues turn so deep a brown that they change to a coal-black. The color under the tongue becomes a blackish purple, because the fire element burns so fiercely in the stomach that the inflammation extends even to the kidneys. Many people are skeptical regarding the significance of a coated tongue. However, great suffering can be prevented if people will but watch their tongues closely and take treatment at the very beginning. The different colors also influence the desires and preferences of the different races. For instance, the African-American people like red; the Chinese like yellow and light red; the Caucasian people like white. Likewise, in the human system, because the spleen and the stomach belong to the earth element, they naturally crave sweets and things of yellow coloring.

Consequently, if a person whose spleen is affected is sad and down- hearted, a bouquet of yellow flowers would be a good gift for him. In case a person has heart trouble or his mind is affected, dark blue or dark green would be the most suitable colors for his environment, in order to overcome the fire element.

The five tastes represent the five elements in nature

1. A pungent taste influences the action of the lungs, which belong to the mineral element.
2. A sour taste has power to contract the air in the blood and to assist in the functioning of the gall bladder and liver, which belong to the vegetation element.
3. A bitter taste rushes through the system and works especially upon the heart, which belongs to the fire element.
4. A sweet taste belongs to the earth element; anything sweet has a special effect upon the stomach and spleen.
5. A salty taste belongs to the water element. In nature, the water of the ocean is salty. In the human body, the kidneys and their sub organ, the bladder, belong to the water element. Anything that is salty affects these organs. In the early dawn of Chinese civilization, the Chinese classified all things in nature under the five principal elements. The five tastes are just as important as the five colors or the five musical tones. If a person understands these five tastes, he can tell approximately how any given food will affect his system. If any food has a deleterious effect upon any part' of his system, he can easily abstain from that sort of food.

Of the five tastes, the most destructive to the human system is the bitter (or hot), because it influences the blood passing through the heart.

Chinese theories regarding the heart

The sketch of a heart that is just of like many similar sketches that appeared about three centuries ago in a revised edition of The Encyclopedia of Herbal Science published by the Chinese Imperial College in Peking, China. It shows how the various parts of the body are affected by the different organs and it also shows the connection of the blood vessels with the heart.

Although thousands of years have elapsed since the original of the Chinese sketch was made by eminent herbalists in China, yet great numbers of sufferers from heart trouble in the United States as well as in the Orient are daily obtaining great benefit from this ancient Chinese knowledge by using the Chinese herbal remedies. The heart, which is red like the sun, is classified under the fire element.

When the five principal elements are working with equal balance and power the heart is free from disease. The two main causes of disease of the heart are inflammation and weakness of the heart.

If the blood of the heart is inflamed, it causes high blood pressure and enlargement of the heart, in which latter case the heart swells, cracks and leaks. Inflammation produces pain, gas, palpitation, sore chest, shortness of breath, hardening of the arteries, angina pectoris, swollen legs, dropsy, fits, nervousness, headache, fatigue after slight exertion, a pounding noise in the heart, insanity and heart failure.

According to the Chinese theories, insanity and fits belong to the same class of ailments, the only difference being that one is more violent than the other. Inflammation of the heart and nerves which run from it to the brain is the cause in both cases. The inflammation condenses the moisture, which is the reason why most of the people who have it foam at the mouth. Inflammation of the heart sometimes extends to the small intestines and causes them to bleed. This is the blood that appears in the urine.

Weakness and inflammation combined cause blood clots in the eyes. Such cases frequently baffle the eye specialists. Weakness of the heart sometimes causes one to be afraid of the dark or to fear that someone is plotting to kill him. Such sufferers cry out, lament or have disturbing dreams.

When the heart is weak it causes low blood pressure, paleness, swollen legs, dropsy, etc. A case of sudden fright affects the heart and requires immediate attention. Slight indigestion will cause gas and palpitation of the heart temporarily, but is insufficient cause for alarm.

Each herbalist has his own methods of compounding herbs. The herbs prepared for heart trouble by the herbal specialist cannot be obtained elsewhere. While the herbs in these compounds are mild and harmless, yet they are effective.

How to care for the heart-natures way

Just as the sun is the fire element of nature, so is the heart the fire element of the human body. Of all the elements, the fire element is the most active. A sudden shock has a more noticeable effect upon the heart than upon any of the other organs, When the blood, the muscle of the valve of the heart, or the heart itself is inflamed or is overtaxed because of exertion or sudden fright the heart beats fast. Pain, leakage or rush of blood to the head may ensue. Physicians have termed the latter "high blood pressure." It is variously accompanied by gas, dizziness, sleeplessness, difficult breathing, paralytic stroke, etc.

Chinese theories regarding the lungs

The lungs as belonging to the mineral element. Just as the heart controls the blood circulation, the lungs control the air circulation of the human system. If the blood of the lungs is in good condition, and the pores of the body are kept clean, while at the same time the lungs are free from inflammation, impurities, and abnormal temperature of foreign origin, the lungs are strong and healthy.

Herbs of white color and of either pungent or insipid taste belong to the mineral element. The former cause the heat of the body to expand and to go down to the limbs and pass outward through the skin. The activity of the lungs extends also to the sub-organs and the intestines. The herbs of insipid taste free the lungs and intestines of fever.

The common cold

When one has a cold in any part or in the whole of the body, the passages of the pores are closed. As the internal heat cannot then escape, it forces its way up to the head, which begins to ache. If this heat (fever) reaches the lungs, pneumonia may result. When a cold settles in any part of the body, it stops the circulation both of the blood and of the air in that part. Stiff neck and pain in the follow. The internal fever causes a dryness and a soreness of the throat. If the heat in the lungs interferes with the free passage of the air, there is coughing.

For these reasons, a herb compound for a cold generally contains more than a dozen different kinds of herbs, such as : Herbs to take away the fever from the lungs; herbs to open the passages of the pores, so that the lungs and pores may work again in unison; herbs to soothe the air passages of the bronchial tubes; herbs to pacify the blood of the liver; herbs to carry away the feverish congestion, so that the head will stop aching. A herb compound for a cold is therefore much more beneficial than any sort of drugs. This is the reason why Chinese herbalists have been so successful in relieving cases of the common cold and also Influenza.

Eczema connected to the health of the lungs

A certain class of skin disease is commonly known as Eczema. Because the pores of the skin work in unison with the lungs, germs and impurities in the skin and pores affect the blood, through the medium of the lungs, to a greater or less degree. Consequently, herbs for Eczema must be so compounded as to remove the impurities from the blood, through the action of the lungs, which will drive out the impurities through the pores. In addition to this, herb salve or herb powder is generally applied externally. Herbs are also boiled for washing the affected parts.

When disease affects either the lower or the upper limbs, herbs for cleansing the spleen must be added to the herbs in the compound for the lungs, as the spleen controls the limbs. Although Eczema and other skin diseases are disagreeable, they are not dangerous.

Asthma due to the lungs

When a chronic cold settles in the lungs, they become clogged with mucous congestion. This condition is known as Asthma. If the case is of long standing, the sufferer's health is gradually impaired, and it requires considerable time to restore it to normal. An good Chinese herbalist has a splendid record for the absolute and permanent relief of Asthma cases.

Throat diseases

When equilibrium of power and balance is maintained in the working of the five elements, the human system is free from disease. The throat is a narrow passage between the trunk of the body and the head. In it are numerous small nerves and glands which connect with the internal organs such as the lungs, kidneys, stomach, liver, and heart.

The lungs as well as the kidneys help clean the blood is so thoroughly cleansed that there is no congestion, and the pores function freely. In consequence, if this state of balance is maintained you will rarely catches cold.

The Chinese herbs for a cold are beneficial to the entire system, and are very different from the treatments prescribed by other schools of healing, in which alcoholic liquor is often used. The fever or inflammation in the system is thus augmented instead of being driven out. Herbs for colds also tend to drive away Influenza germs, just as tobacco plants keep insects away from the garden, and tobacco smoke keeps away snakes.

Sinus problems- The causes and symptoms

According to Chinese Theories, sinus trouble is attributable to the following causes:

1. The nose is the cavity of the lungs. If a cold is contracted, the heat (fever) centers in the head and lungs.
2. The mouth is the cavity to the stomach. If a person either eats too frequently or if he eats too much spicy, fried, greasy or rich food, there will be a certain amount of indigestion in the stomach, and the blood there will become heated. Naturally, as the blood circulates and the air passes out and upward from the lungs and the stomach, the sinus is liable to become affected. If the sinus is painful and the mucus is thick, yellowish brown, and if dry discharges come from the nose, it indicates that one has heated blood in the lungs and perhaps more or less indigestion. It also indicates that there is too much of the fire element in the blood.

If the mucus discharged through the nose is clear, thin, and abundant, and if these discharges are sometimes accompanied by pain, a severe chronic cold has settled in the head and has concentrated in the sinus. When a person has chronic sinus trouble, his health is often impaired and there is an unpleasant odor about his nose or mouth. The entire system is sometimes poisoned, and in severe cases of sinus trouble, the nose swells painfully.

Because of the Chinese method of healing with herbs, many operations have been avoided. There are two methods of compounding herbs for sinus trouble. One is to use herbs to purify the blood of the stomach and lungs and to dispel the heat, combined with herbs to improve the digestion and to open the passages or cavities of the sinus. The other method is to use herbs to clear out the cold and to restore the blood strength, so that relief may be permanent. If a person is weak and the sinus trouble of long standing, a considerable length of time may be required.

Chinese theories regarding the liver an gall bladder

The sketch reproduced here is one of many similar sketches that appeared about three centuries ago in a revised edition of the Encyclopedia of Herbal Science, published by the Chinese Imperial College in Peking, China. It shows how the various nerves in different parts of the body are affected by the gall bladder and liver. Although thousands of years have elapsed since the original of the accompanying sketch was made by eminent herbalists in China, yet great numbers of sufferers from liver and gall bladder trouble in the U. S. as well as in Asia are daily obtaining great benefit from this ancient Chinese knowledge by using the Chinese herbal remedies. Because the liquid in the gall bladder and the juices secreted by the liver are greenish, thus resembling the vegetation element in color,

The ancient Chinese concluded that the gall bladder and liver belonged to the vegetation element and that herbs of green color and sour taste should be used as correctives for disorders of these organs. Upon experimenting, he discovered that herbs of this sort have power to contract the air in the blood, and that their action assists the liver and gall bladder in functioning.

The liver acts as a reservoir to hold the blood until it is thrown back into circulation. The secretions of the liver and gall bladder enter the intestines and aid digestion. The gall bladder is a sub-organ to the liver. The inflamed condition of the liver causes inflammation and congestion of the Gall Duct; and the Bile either overflows, causing Yellow Jaundice or solidifies into Gallstones. At intervals the Liver becomes greatly inflamed, causing swelling in the entire right side of the trunk, from the glands of the neck to the lower part of the abdomen. The Appendix then swells and Appendicitis sets in. When the stones are passing through, they cause such intense pain that the sufferer frequently loses consciousness. As a symptom of Gall and Liver Troubles there is generally more or less pain, starting beneath the right rib and running around the right side, up to the shoulder blades.

If either the liver or gall bladder is inflamed or is weak and in-active, pain, enlargement, gall stones, biliousness, sleeplessness, nervousness, discoloration of the skin and a ringing or buzzing noise in the ears may follow. Sometimes, when the inflammation is severe, it causes running sores or even ulcers in the ears, deafness, inflamed eyes, blindness, hot flashes or headaches. Intense anger also affects the liver. Protracted sorrow causes the liver to be sluggish and the blood to become poisoned. This condition is favorable to the formation of growths, especially in the breast.

Americans physicians often laugh at the Chinese idea that the liver is partly on the left side of the body as well as on the right. Through their studies, the Chinese have found that the pulse of the circulation of the liver is determined by feeling the pulse in the left wrist, instead of in the right.

When through fright, anger or other strong emotion, the liver is stimulated abnormally, it gets into a fiery condition. The individual is then liable to be quick-tempered, to talk fast and loud, or if in pain, to groan or cry in a loud voice. An abnormally active liver frequently deprives one of the use of his voice entirely for a short period of time.

This is why certain persons often find it necessary to stop and rest for a time before going on with a speech at a public meeting, or continuing in a private discussion. The presence of fever in the liver cannot be detected by the thermometer used by the medical profession, but must be discovered in other ways. The Chinese herbs for the liver act independently through the blood circulation. Generally, it is not necessary to physic through the bowels. Cleansing the liver by physic is an Occidental method. When an adult or child is suffering, if he groans or cries continuously, with a loud, steady voice,

The Liver and Gall Bladder there is no doubt that he has inflammation of the liver and adjacent organs.

The liver is one of the five principal organs, the gall bladder being one of its sub-organs. Pain in the right side, the region of the liver, is generally caused by inflammation of that organ or by the secretions of the liver overflowing into the gall bladder, where they either become bile or solidify into stones. Physicians frequently cut out either the gall bladder or the appendix. They prefer not to cut out the main organ, the liver, because that operation would be both dangerous and difficult. Consequently, the liver is generally left untouched and many persons whose gall bladders have been removed still suffer considerable pain in the right side and lie in bed for years.

According to Chinese theories, the liver controls the nerves. When there is rheumatic nerve trouble, attention must be given to the liver, and herbs must also be added to the compound to drive out the accumulated poison.

How Chinese herbs combat disease

Chinese Herbs properly compounded to combat disease may be compared to an army organized to attack an enemy. The Herbalist is the Commander; his Knowledge, Experience, Intelligence, and Astuteness are the Spies. In order to detect an ailment, the Herbalist must use his eyes in studying the skin of the sufferer, just as the Aviator must use his eyes in locating the enemy and in discovering his strong and weak points.

When an army is very strong and powerful, in order to defeat it, the attacking force must secure other nations as allies. Likewise, in overcoming serious ailments, it requires the combined powers of a number of varieties of herbs, all working together in harmonious alliance, to eradicate the disease.

The kidneys and bladder

About 300 years ago, a sketch was revised and published in the Encyclopedia of Herbal Science by the Chinese Imperial College in Peking, China. It shows every point at which the nerves are affected by the kidneys and their sub-organ, the bladder. Numerous ills are caused by the im- proper functioning of these organs. In order to reach the seat of these diseases, one must have both a knowledge of herbal compounds and of the ancient Chinese theories of anatomy with regard to these organs. Although the original of the accompanying sketch was made by eminent herbalists in China, thousands of years ago, the herbalists of today can still learn from it. However, just as there are differences in intelligence, so are there differences in herbalists. To eliminate doubt, people should consult A scholarly and reliable herbalist.

In the beginning of Chinese civilization, there was an emperor known as Shin Nong. He not only classified the herbs under five natural elements, according to their color and taste, but he also classified the five vital organs of the body under the five principal elements.

1. The stomach is yellow like the earth.

2 . The heart is red like the sun.
3 . The kidneys are dark colored like the ocean water.
4 . The lungs are white like the minerals.
5 . The secretions of the liver are greenish like vegetation.

Each of these organs has related organs. The kidneys are those organs of the human system that resemble the water in the ocean. They distribute nourishment through the body by means of the nerves. The nerves of the lower limbs come through the kidneys and pass up the back, through the neck, and over the head and eyes. All these nerves depend on the kidneys for their strength and nourishment, just like the earth depends on the water element of the oceans for its rains and moisture.

When the kidneys fail to function properly because of inflammation, or by reason of weakness, they become the source of numerous ailments. In case of inflammation, people sometimes have Slight's disease, floating kidneys, etc. The tendency of inflammation (the fire element) is to cause swelling, especially of the lower limbs, which frequently develops into dropsy. Sometimes inflammation of the kidneys causes the lower limbs to cramp. This is accompanied by burning pain from the small of the back down to the toes, and is commonly known as Rheumatism, or Neuritis. When it gets a strong and lasting grip, the sufferer is crippled for life.

Inflammation of the kidneys also causes constipation, because it dries up the moisture of the blood circulation in the bowels. In inflammation of the kidneys, or prostatic trouble, the urine is dark colored, and there is frequent voiding of small quantities.

In cases where kidneys are weak and inactive, they cause dizziness, weakness, backache, headache, stiffness and pain in the back of the neck, which continues up into the nerves of the head, ringing or buzzing noises in the ear and even cross eyes. This condition is accompanied by loss of vitality, forgetfulness, brain fatigue, poor concentration and shortness of breath and frequent voiding of large quantities of urine.

In a person who is consumptive or in one who coughs frequently for other reasons, the lungs become dry and feverish, and the kidneys are therefore liable to become inflamed. When these organs do not function in unison, a condition sets in that is difficult to relieve. The liver, stomach and spleen become affected one after the other, the spleen being the last to become diseased. When the spleen is affected, the sufferer has then but a week or two live!

The Kidneys

The herbs for the restoration of the kidneys to normal are of various kinds. Each compound for a cup of tea contains from 13 to 20 different kinds of herbs. If the kidneys are inflamed, two or three varieties of herbs are put in to bring them plenty of good blood; two or three kinds to accumulate more moisture in the kidneys; two or three kinds to cause the moisture or water to flush the kidneys; one or two kinds to work through the nerves to the lower limbs and upper parts of the body; one kind to work into the lungs, from which the kidneys gain part of their strength, and motive power; one kind to purify and cleanse the bladder, and one kind to clean out the liver and cool the blood.

The number of packages of these herbs necessary to bring permanent relief depends upon the severity of the ailment and length of time it has persisted. Generally, the herb compound must be changed as the condition of the kidneys change. When herbs are compounded for weakness of the kidneys, very different herbs are given from those required for inflammation. Many persons try to get relief by merely flushing the kidneys with water without the addition of any curative elements. The result is often the overburdening of the kidneys, and the weakening of the bladder. Furthermore, the drinking of too much water causes indigestion, and sooner or later the health of the individual is broken by dilution.

The change of life in man (andropause)

While most people are familiar with the term "Change of Life" as applied to woman, few realize that man also undergoes a change of life. For thousands of years the Chinese people have been taught that the life of both sexes is divided into periods of time, or cycles. A woman's life is divided into cycles of 7 years. The first cycle is that of early childhood; at the close of the second cycle, she is 14 years of age, and has developed into young womanhood. When she has completed 7 cycles of 7 years each, the average woman has come to the change of life, although she is but 49 years of age.

With man, each cycle consists of 8 years instead of 7 years. He develops into young manhood at the age of 16 years, after having completed two cycles of 8 years each. Moreover, he must complete 8 cycles of 8 years duration before he comes to the change of life, at which time he is therefore 64 years of age.

Because of this difference in the age at which men and women reach the change of life, we may infer that a man who is 15 years older than his wife is actually of the same age physiologically, and that though younger in years, a wife who is less than 15 years younger than her husband is really the elder of the two.

During the period of their change of life, most men suffer because of difficulties in the functioning of the kidneys and bladder, accompanied by more or less dizziness of the head and pain in the back of the neck, etc. This trouble may be traced to the loss of power by the kidneys, due to the change of life in man. When, from about 55 to 65 years of age, many suffering men consult their physicians regarding these ailments, the physicians generally diagnose the trouble as swollen glands or decide that it is the neck of the bladder that is causing the trouble.

Frequently the bladder is operated upon and left leaky as long as the man lives. However, the real seat of the trouble is to be found in the change of life, which has lessened the power of the kidneys, thus weakening the circulation of the blood and the air pressure.

Fortunately many herbs and combination of herbs are able to help with this condition. The key is to always “cycle” on and off the herbs for a period of 6-8 weeks. Some of these herbs are; Hou Shu wu (Fo-Ti), ginseng (all vanities) , snake root, saw palmetto berry, maca root, Tong kat ali, and many more. See-“Glossary of herbs”.

Healthy teeth and gums

It is a great blessing to have good, sound teeth, it is a calamity not to have them. For thousands of years, the Chinese Theories have shown that the hair is a part of the blood and that the teeth are a part of the bones. Hence, because the bones are controlled by the kidneys, the teeth are also controlled by them.

If one's vital organs, the heart, the liver, the intestines, the gall bladder, the stomach, the spleen, the kidneys, and the lungs, are functioning properly and in unison and are free from inflammation, there is no reason why he should have either toothache or decayed teeth.

From very ancient times, the Chinese Herbalists have been agreed in attributing tooth troubles to the eight following causes :

1. Pain in the upper incisors is caused by the fire element of the heart.
2. Pain in the upper cuspids and bicuspids is caused by the fire element of the stomach.
3. Pain in the lower incisors is caused by the fire element of the kidneys.
4. Pain in the lower cuspids and bicuspids is caused by the fire element of the spleen.
5. Pain in the upper left molars is caused by the fire element of the large intestines.
6. Pain in the upper right molars is caused by the fire elements of the gall bladder.
7. Pain in the lower left molars is caused by the fire element of the lungs.
8. Pain in the lower right molars is caused by the fire element of the liver.

One who suffers from toothache should secure immediate relief from the inflammation of the internal organs before decay sets in or the gums become ulcerated. Usually, a person with a sore gum consults a medical man and is advised by him to see a dentist and either have his teeth extracted or certain drugs injected to deaden the nerves or the roots of the teeth. If the natural teeth are extracted and false teeth fitted, the food is thereafter either only partially chewed or not masticated at all. Indigestion and failing health result.

A case in point is that of a man who suffered so severely with toothache that he was unable to eat. He therefore called upon a dentist to find out whether his teeth were decaying. The dentist informed him that all his teeth were in good condition and that there was no sign of decay, but that the gum around one tooth had grown up higher than the tooth, and was, therefore, bitten between the two teeth whenever the mouth was closed, thus causing pain.

The sufferer then called upon the herbalist, who asked him how long he had suffered with the pain. The reply was : "About a week." Now the herbalist immediately realized that as the sufferer had a gum in his mouth ever since he was born, which was over 35 years, there was no reason for it to suddenly "grow up" in a week. He therefore prepared a cup of tea to subdue the fire element in the man's stomach. The sufferer drank the tea at 5 p. m. and the next morning he found that the swelling and soreness had all gone out of his gum.

Many persons, after either having their teeth filled or plates made by a good dentist, still find their gums sore and raw at times. Then they mistakenly blame the dentist because they think that their fillings were not properly put in or that their false teeth are not a good fit, when, in fact, the real cause of the rawness and soreness of their gums is traceable to internal disorders.

People without teeth

With the hope of gaining relief, approximately 80% of people who are sick have their teeth extracted. Unfortunately, however, their ills continue. Throughout his long period of experience, herbalists have found that, due to the lack of a fundamental knowledge of the human system, a great many people have acted upon the merciless advice that they have either part or all of their good teeth extracted. This has been done notwithstanding the fact that these persons were suffering from Neuritis, Rheumatism, Headache, or from some other nervous derangement that had absolutely no connection with the teeth, but was caused by the improper functioning of one or more of the internal organs of the body. Not realizing that their pain was due to inflammation of and impurities in their blood, caused by this non-functioning, these people have mistakenly placed too much faith in blood tests, which, by microscopic or other methods, show germs of disease only, but do not show blood impurities, poison, or inflammation. Even the health of the teeth and gums depends upon the condition of the blood. Because persons with artificial teeth cannot chew well, they get but a portion of the value of the food with which to nourish their bodies. Their health is generally rated as "Third Class" and they have soreness of the gums which frequently causes them to go without their teeth. It is pitiful to see a grown person with a mouth like that of a toothless infant.

Herbs have not only cleansed the systems of many persons, afflicted with various ills, but they have also helped to eradicate pyorrhea and to heal diseased gums. In addition to herbs you should massage your gums gently everyday this applies to both tooth-less people and if you still have your teeth. Use both your fingers and toothbrush at least 3 times per day.

Chinese theories regarding rheumatism, paralysis, neuritis, and convulsions.

These ailments originate from similar causes and belong to the same family of diseases. Rheumatism is the more common of the five. The Chinese characters for Rheumatism are "Fung Sep," which mean "Wind and Dampness." The Chinese attribute this disease to four causes :

1. To the air circulation in the body. The "Fung" (wind) circulates in the body just as the air circulates in space. If the air circulation is impeded, it becomes wind of certain velocity. The wind causes pain to move from one part of the body to another.
2. To dampness. The dampness in the body resembles the dampness or moisture in the air. If the dampness is heavy, it causes dull, heavy pain in the human body.
3. To inflammation. Inflammation in the body is like the heat waves that cause lightning, storms, etc., on the earth. Inflammation swells the tissues and causes pain.
4. To cold. The cold or chilliness in the body resembles the cold or chill ("Hon" in Chinese) of the earth. It causes excruciatingly sharp, shooting pains, especially in the hips and legs.

In the case of a rheumatic sufferer, more than one, and sometimes all four of these causes are operative to a greater or less degree. Ninety percent of the sufferers from rheumatism have kidney and bladder troubles, which weaken the nerves and the blood circulation. Wind, dampness, inflammation and cold are liable to affect the body both from internal and external sources. Unless one's blood circulation is ir reparably deteriorated, the correct herbs will eradicate the causes of Rheumatism.

Although Rheumatism may come on either suddenly or gradually, paralysis generally comes on suddenly. Paralysis may affect but one side of the human body or one or more of the limbs. Paralysis is un-accompanied by pain, and the affected part becomes somewhat like a piece of rubber hose, entirely devoid of feeling. Attacks of paralysis are generally due to the improper functioning of the stomach and lungs, together with an affection of the nerves. Paralysis is often combined with Rheumatism.

Neuritis is both painful and very common, but it is not dangerous.

A Convulsion is a spell of nervous attack. While it causes severe pain, it seldom causes death. Herbalist's have relieved numerous cases of Neuritis and of Convulsions.

Apoplexy is more dangerous than Rheumatism, Neuritis, Paralysis, or Convulsion. A sudden and severe attack of Apoplexy causes instant death. If the stricken one has lockjaw and his fist is closed tight, there is hope for his recovery. If his mouth is wide open, it shows that his heart is failing. If his eyes are closed, his liver is failing. If his hands are open, his spleen is failing. If he voids urine, his kidney strength is gone. Sometimes the face of the sufferer is blood red and the sweat pours out. Any of these terrible symptoms show that there is no hope. Many apoplectic's who have survived slight attacks have been left with a wryness of the mouth, or have lost their voices or the use of one or more of their limbs.

Chinese theories regarding the blood

The blood is the vital fluid that circulates through the arteries and veins of the human system. By reason of the derangement of one or all of the vital organs, the blood becomes poisoned through infection, inflammation, or contagion. Impurities in the blood often cause eruptions to appear on the skin in different parts of the body. Microscopic tests of the blood show various figures and signs of lymphatic infection, and the results of blood tests are often reported as from one to three plus positive. When this is the case, the sufferer frequently becomes worried and downhearted. Many such have taken dozens of hypodermic injections and have been under the treatment of medical men for years, yet their blood tests still show X's, or one to three plus positive. To obtain permanent relief is a hard problem.

According to the Chinese theories, there are two classes of sufferers from blood disorders, for each of which a different method of treatment should be employed.

First, if a person infected with poisonous inflammation has

robust health, the treatment should be a compound of herbs to cool the blood, thus eliminating the inflammation, and of herbs to cleanse all the internal organs.

If eruptions occur in certain parts of the body, some herbs should be put into the compound to reach those places through the vital organs. Anyone who faithfully gives his body a chance to get clean always succeeds.

Second, if a person has chronic lymphatic infection and is in a weakened condition, the compound should contain herbs to rebuild the entire system and insure the proper functioning of all vital organs. Herbs should also be added to expel the impurities through the air and blood circulations, especially to drive the impurities out through the pores, thus helping the lungs in their work. It takes much longer to over- come the trouble when the sufferer is in a chronic, weakened condition, than when he is strong. Many persons seek to drive out the infection by taking repeated doses of physic, but the result is only to weaken the blood circulation and to permit the infection to become more deeply rooted.

The best time to shave

The human body is like an engine. When an engine has run continuously for any length of time, it is liable to become overheated. The body of a person who has worked all day likewise becomes overheated. Some men shave early in the morning, while others shave either in the evenings or at any time during the day. Those who suffer either from sore chins or from "Barbers' Itch" should try shaving the first thing in the morning, at which time the blood is cool and the skin is firm and taut. Therefore, one who shaves in the morning not only gets a cleaner, closer shave, but his skin is less easily inflamed.

However, men who patronize the barbers need not be particular about being shaved so early in the day, as conditions at the barbers are somewhat different, and the following benefits are obtainable:

1. As one rests and relaxes in the barber's chair, the blood cools.
2. The barber's razor is generally sharper than that of the individual; therefore, a clean shave is obtained with fewer strokes.
3. The barber takes his time, while the individual is often in a hurry. When one is hurried, the razor is not only liable to slip but the blood is almost certain to became inflamed, thus making a close shave well-nigh impossible.

The Herbalist always advises such patrons to shave early in the morning, in case they do their own shaving. Those who have followed this advice have obtained speedy results. This is one reason 'after-shave' was invented with alcohol to sooth minute cuts that even if no bleeding is detected the skin (and therefore your first barrier of protection from infection) has been compromised and allow a few hours to buildup a healing over the face. Which is also know due to its proximity to the heart and brain (blood flow) to be the fastest healing (and bleeding) areas of the human body.

How herbs stop pain without drugs

Chinese Herbs stop pain by eradicating the following causes:

1. Poisonous inflammation causes congestion of the blood in one place, which then either begins to swell or to form a cancer. This causes great pain. After the blood has been cleansed by the herbs, the inflammation subsides and the pain stops.
2. In a cancer sufferer whose blood circulation is poor, the cancer is slow to develop, and the pain becomes intense at night. When the person is walking or keeps moving, the pain is greatly lessened. In cases of this kind, the blood should be enriched and strengthened with nourishing herbs, combined with herbs to free the blood of poisonous substances. Then the cancer or growth will develop quickly and come out. In this way, pain is overcome by Chinese Herbal Remedies without resort to Cocaine, Morphine, or any other drug.

Chinese theories regarding cancer

For thousands of years, the Chinese have believed that Cancers are caused by inflammation and by poison in the blood. When any of the five vital organs of the body fails to function properly, the blood in that organ becomes poison, and heat is generated the same as when a volcano eruption occurs on the earth. Therefore, when a cancer is formed anywhere in the body, there must be something wrong with one or more of the vital organs.

According to the Chinese definition, the difference between a tumor and a cancer is that the former is a growth located inside the body, which cannot be seen from the outside, while a cancer is a growth that forms beneath the skin and develops above the skin, its size being an inch or more in diameter. When a cancer forms in a neck gland, it has originated from the blood of the liver.

Breast cancer in women is due to poison in the spleen which affects the milk glands, because women are liable to periods of sadness, worry and melancholy. (Also now it can be traced directly to women who place their cellular phones in their bra and or 'tex' and talk for long periods f time) Cancer of the internal ovaries (and other sex organs) may be traced to the improper functioning of the bladder and kidneys.

Canker sores and boils in the mouth are due to impure blood in the stomach because the mouth is the outer cavity of the stomach.

The air and the blood circulations cause soreness to be exposed in the mouth and also by a red, sore nose, by boils, on the nose or by hemorrhoids, because the nose is the cavity of the lungs. If the blood or the air in the lungs is impure, or if there is too much fire (inflammation) these maladies of the nose are caused. When hemorrhoids, or sores, or noises are located in the ears, they are due to improper functioning or to impure blood in the liver and kidneys, because, according to Chinese theories, the ears are the cavities of the liver and kidneys. Inflammation of the rectum, piles or fistulas are due to the large intestines and the lungs, as the large intestines are the sub-organs to the lungs. When eruptions or itches appear on the skin on the upper part of the body, blood purifiers are necessary for the lungs, which control the pores of the body. Certain cancers may be easily overcome before they spread and eat into the tissues. However, there is no help if they are allowed to go until the tissues are consumed, for a fireman cannot save a house that is already burned to the ground.

Chinese methods of prevention and healing

When a cancer begins, it commences to swell, to have pain and fever, and to form lumps. At this stage, according to Chinese theories if the herbs are compounded to cleanse the blood of the vital organs, and external applications are made, the cancer will generally disappear.

In a case, however, where cancer has not been completely eradicated before being formed, herbs must be compounded to cause the blood circulation to force the poison to collect at the spot where external treatments can draw it to a head, and help it to ripen, and to break out.

The Chinese do not believe, as do the Americans, in the possibility of discovering some one thing, such as serum, gamma rays, X-Rays, or application of electricity to cure all kinds of cancer, regardless of location, whether on the head, the rectum, or the mouth. Numerous cancers, where X-Rays, electricity, or other methods have been used, the result is that the flesh has been baked into hard chunks of poisoned flesh. The cancer keeps right on growing underneath this big chunk of flesh, and the condition is a thousand times harder to relieve.

Scientists are continually making new inventions and discoveries, but the members of the medical profession in no part of the world have discovered anything to cure cancer. They have become afraid of it and have had a law passed forbidding anyone to advertise a cancer cure. Some of the large dailies even refuse to print the word cancer in their sheets. Thus, is knowledge of how to gain relief in case of cancer kept away from the people. Although for fifty centuries China has had numerous books which have taught the people how to cope with various ailments, including cancer, still ,in the case of the latter, further research was necessary.

About three hundred years ago, a kind-hearted Emperor summoned the herbalists from all over the country to a great conference. Among them were several hundred who had passed the Imperial Examinations with the first and second degrees. As a result of the conference and the diligence of these scholarly herbalists, a great work of twenty volumes was compiled to be used as textbooks on the healing of dis- ease by the government and people. This work gives clear instructions regarding all kinds of cases, but it takes an intelligent, experienced herbalist, with an extensive knowledge in the dispensing of herbs to secure results, as the system of each individual sufferer differs in strength and each case has its own complications.

Dangerous tanning-beds and taking a sunbath

The secret of the Chinese methods of healing is the bringing of the elements of the human body to function properly and evenly. In other words keeping in 'balance' all things. When it is dark in the winter months, then instead of seeking artificial sunlight in the form of the toxic tanning-beds. You should instead give your body what it is craving without damaging your skin. This is vitamin D3! You can take anywhere from 5,000 -20,000 I.U.s of this amazing vitamin during the winter months. Your energy and spirit should return to normal.

During the spring and summer months you should then discontinue the Vitamin D3 and enjoy the sun on your skin's surface. Lay outside in the nude or as little clothing as possible anywhere from 15 minutes to an hour will provide your body with natural Vitamin D much like a plant makes sugars and starches via photosynthesis. Your body when exposed to sunlight will manufacture Vitamin D and increase your health and healing many times over. Take care as not to over indulge in the sun for hours as you may become sunburned and this is not good for your health.

Another Vitamin that should be included is Vitamin C. This miraculous vitamin should be taken year round. The average mammalian makes approximately 4,000 milligrams of Vitamin C per day in their own body! This occur's in your average pet dog, to a mighty tiger in the jungle. However, mankind has lost(or never had) the ability to manufacture

Vitamin C. Unlike Vitamin D which humans can still make with the much needed sunlight. Vitamin C must be taken in either fruits and vegetables or a direct supplement.

I would recommend between 4,000-6,000 milligrams of Vitamin C per day. 4,000 milligrams is the threshold of clearing your blood of all toxic chemicals, boosting your immune system, increasing your I.Q., and prevents cancer!

These effects begin within minutes of taken this Vitamin C and will keep working throughout the day. It is a cheap cost effective supplement that should be added to everyone's diet.

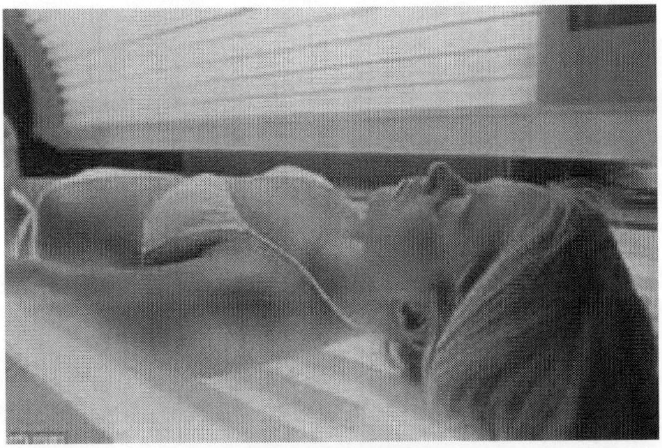

Always a bad idea!

Our sun provides more than enough radiation.

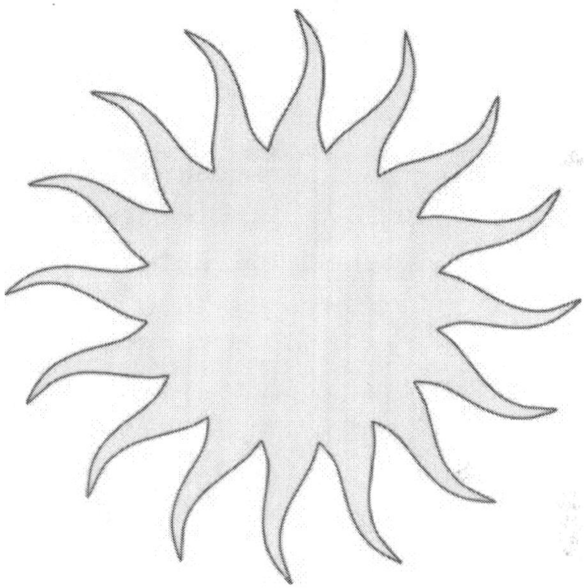

Fake powers

Martial artists are like most people in respect to the wanting to believe in some higher power, or magic. It simply is not out there. The hope, and faith of people keeps them going marching on like mindless wonders sometimes. This unfortunately is where the con-artists and charlatans come into play.

When people that are unfamiliar with the unknown such as death of a loved one or friend. They become very susceptible to so-called spiritualist, mediums, necromancer's, etc. that 'prey' on the victims misery even more by charging them money in exchange for a hope of communication with the dearly departed. Why this occurs so frequently and now even on televised regular programing. Is the hunger from being suddenly cut off (communication) from the dearly departed. The pain of this is often so strong that common sense is not used. Instead people go with the emotion's (which are so often still charged) making them even more vulnerable to believing in the fake-medium relating the 'already known' information gained from newspaper's, library's, and now the internet, combined with the 'soft-touch' interrogation techniques they all use, when speaking with the loved one that is still in highly emotional state of loss. In fact not one of these so-called mediums use any other question's and answer's back and forth dialog. It is the same exact series of 'fishing for known answer's' any competent interrogator has used.

The great Magician Harry Houdini (Ehric Weiss) traveled around the country and uncovered the fakes duping people out of money for years. He did a great credit by removing the superstitious fraudulent criminals, an yet still to this day, people want to believe in something that does not exist. The human emotional often overwhelms the logical common sense part of our mind. Not because we are weak, but because the alternative is unbearable. So, to keep the 'hope' alive the fake mediums still keep taking good emotionally scared people's money.

The same is often true with martial artists. Many colorful legend's are passed down through centuries of story telling both written and oral. These wonderful tales, have caught the hear of most martial artists at one time or another.

However, this same gullibility of wanting to believe in something that is not there, again often overwhelms the rational thinking and succumbs to fanciful tales of legends. True, most legends are based on a glimmer of truth, that has been distorted over time by either design or misinterpretation. One such 'power' is the ability to not be hurt by extreme temperatures. I recall a street demonstration in Hong Kong (after being asked to stop and watch) as a martial art's 'Master' and I use this word loosely. Looked at the bubbling pot of hot oil and thrust his hand into it without showing any discomfort and kept in the 'hot oil bath' for a minute.

Withdrawing his hand and wiping it off to the applause of the stopped tourists. Then smiling holding out a hat for money. Which I tossed in a few coins along with other on lookers. I even managed to shake the 'Master's' hand-noting no burn to his skin at all. Asking him how he did this 'trick' he just replied "Ch'i power". Being more practical I went about my shopping with my friends and circled back on the way home. Observing the same 'Master' preforming this trick all day I suppose. This time I saw him preparing the hot oil (which was peanut oil) but in addition to this he poured in some 'BORAX'. This combination will make the oil appear to boil, when in fact it is just a chemical reaction at a much lower temperature than actual boiling oil.

So, for the people not knowing the 'trick' will think that this man has some power that can prevent him from being burned. When in fact it is a simple trick of appearance, and knowledge of basic chemistry.

Now we can look at the physic's of breaking. It does take a lot of practice and discipline to break a wooden board(s), bricks(s), or concrete blocks. I am in no way denying that I have broke many objects with the controlled application of a kick, or hand strike.

However, after 2-3 objects are broken and like I have done added 'spacers' (small pieces of wood or other material) in-between the many blocks or bricks. This breaking force needed to break 9 patio blocks is the same as breaking 2-3 patio blocks. You could add even more an in fact eventually just the slightest direct applied force will break the first few blocks and then the weight and momentum of the structure as a whole will break the rest down to the very bottom.

The 'appearance' is that you just broke 9-10- or 12 patio blocks with a single blow. But the reality is 'if' the patio blocks were placed one directly atop the other, or if it was a solid block of cement 3 feet thick. It is doubtful anyone would be able to break a solid block in this manner.

Sifu Tony Salvitti breaking 9 concrete patio blocks (with spacers)

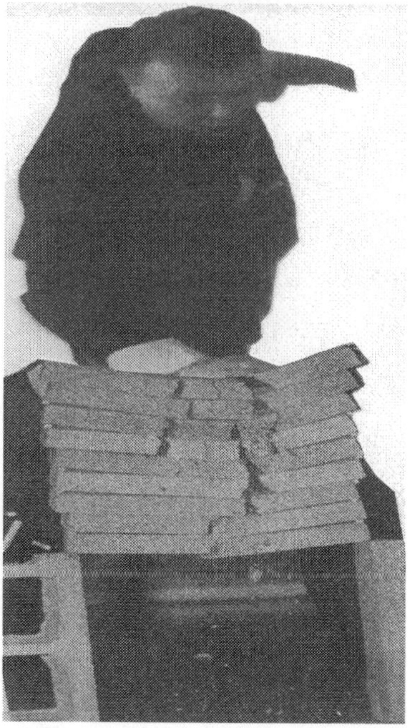

There are many such examples; starting fire without any apparent contact to paper (the use of delayed combustible chemicals is always at hand, moving objects without any apparent means (the use of wires or almost invisible string and or a assistant or magnets-some bricks can have a iron nail deep inside them for this purpose), making water splash and jump out of a bronze pan (these are made with handles on the sides that you or the demonstrator rubs back and forth vigorously and then sets up a standing wave of vibrations that will affect the water or any liquid in the basin).

Some 'powers' are not powers at all but skills developed over many years of practice. To an average person of course the feats that can be accomplished are amazing-but not miraculous!

Another skill that can be developed is speed. Being fast enough to put out a candle with a thrust towards the lit candle without actually touching the flame can be accomplished. This is done with many months to years of diligent drilling and breath control. Eventually you will develop a secondary 'reflex arc' in your neural pathways so you can throw a lightning fast punch without even thinking about it.

The legend around this type of training is something along the lines of; "When you can extinguish a candle from a few feet away, you will be able to best any man or knockout any man". Over the course of centuries colorful legends grew and some small additions made the story more fantastic. Such as; "When you can extinguish the candle from a few feet away you can knock-out or knock-down an opponent without touching him". This small addition has come down in various legends all over Asia.

The fact that you must train throwing hundreds of punches every morning and every evening for ten years or more, keeps the average person from finding out if this is even possible? My own curiosity propelled me to train diligently for over ten years doing this in fact and the ability to snuff out a candle at lightning speed is true and develop a secondary reflex arc as far as kicking and punching ability are true. However, I cannot merely point at a candle and put it out or throw a lightning punch at an opponent and knock him down or out without contact.

Ch'i kung

One of the most important things to learn when first beginning Tai ch'i chuan or any martial art is meditation and breathing. These two things can be done by everyone alive even if you feel you are too old, or handicapped, or paralyzed from the waist down.

This is also the first and last thing you do when you are an accomplished adept at an internal martial art, Hsing-i-chuan and Bau gua being the other two major ones or even just practicing a specialized Ch'i kung (Qi Gong).

In the more advanced stages of this applied self discipline, you can exercise while sitting, or reclined circulating the built up ch'i around your body guided only by your thoughts and will power "wei". This has been called "Kong Jin" and more detailed information is in my original book "Secrets of ch'i kung" about that.

Needless to say you must first have 'something' to circulate. You will need to build up your vital force or ch'i, ki, qi, prana, ka, huna, and many more names all relating to the most abundant energy force in the universe. It is this life force that guides all animated matter and can be used to heal or kill, attract or repulse, begin or end a life.

The scope of this book is to introduce you to being able to generate and control this mysterious life force henceforth referred to as "Ch'i".

Meditation-your first lesson

The only thing that does not belong exclusively to this world is your mind. Our bodies return to te earth from which they were created. But your mind is your consciousness that transcends even death.

Other cultures do not distinguish the mind from the soul or spirit, that occupies the clay vessel you are currently residing in since your conception.

Your mind dictates to your body. This is what you must maintain in order to become a master of it. Not the other way around! So many people (the majority by far) let the body dictate to the mind what is real and what conditions, or diseases you will have to contend with.

It is a fact that over 90% of all Western medical visits are either psychosomatic or require only basic first aid. The fact that physicians in the Western countries are first to whip out the prescription pad and offer drugs. Without even attempting to find the root cause of the problem.

If you control your mind, you can control your body down to every last cell. This is a fact issued by all types of yoga especially Hatha and Raja yoga. It is no mystery that Bodhidharma at Shaolin temple in Honan province, after Bodhidharma, a Buddhist monk from South India, left the court of the Liang emperor Wu in 527, he eventually found himself at the Shaolin Buddhist temple, where he sat facing a wall for nine years, listening to the ants scream (very deep meditation). Legend has it that Bodhidarma's stare was so intense that he burned a hole threw the rock which is still found at the Shaolin temple to this day.

The monks at the temple would fall asleep during meditation due to the weak bodies (from lack of exercise). Bodhidarma then instructed them in slow moving forms of yoga which later became known as Qi-gong (Ch'i kung). Over many years other exercises were added to make once a pure internal art an external fighting one as well. Encompassing all the animal forms and more special skills for self defense like; iron palm, iron finger, dragon claw, etc. These were called 'kungs' or specialized and advanced methods of cultivating both the yin an the yang into one powerful technique. A student would practice his chosen 'kung' for over ten years in order to master it, and continue for life exercising the unique skill he acquired.

In addition to the instruction provided by Bodhidarma, left the Shaolin temple. Thanking everyone there and leaving and iron box. Inside the box was two books; "Marrow Cleansing Classic", and "Muscle Tendon Change Classic" (Yin Jin Jing). The first book "Marrow Cleansing Classic" was stolen by a renegade monk and only speculation as to what happened to it have been shared down through the centuries. The second book-"Muscle Tendon Change Classic" was left in the Shaolin temple and studied completely. The result is that the powerful martial arts were developed from it. This is all due to their possession of this one manuscript.

Mystical exercises (feeling the ch'i)

This "washing of the marrow and muscles" which I learned decades ago from my Master Kwan Li. Took me about ten years just to understand what was happening while I was practicing this exercise.

It is no wonder why most youth decides to learn the fast yang or external, hard arts kick boxing, karate, ju-jitsu, boxing, Wing Chun, etc. To use or be able to effectively defend yourself with Tai Ch'i Chuan, Hsing-I chuan, or Baguazhang (or other "yin", internal, or soft) martial arts. Takes anywhere from five to ten years-depending on the student and teacher of course.

At any rate I was getting "off point". Science has recently provided benefits of exercise and the fact that when you contract multiple time your muscles an pump fresh oxygenating blood into them. These skeletal muscles act as a blood filter and expel waste products and help cleanse your body internally! This is exactly what The Chinese have been doing with ch'i kung (Qi- gong) for over 3,000 years!

Doing these exercises daily over a period of decades not only will enhance your internal organs but your outward appearance will radiate health and power. So, the "fountain of youth" or well-spring of longevity is inside each of us waiting for it to be tapped. To do this you need only two things; desire, and self discipline.

Ch'i and Jing

Ch'i (Ki-Japanese or Prana-Indian), is the life force you need to nurture within you and cultivate it for a long time.

Jing is the application of ch'i to the external world outside of your body. This may seem fantastic bit you an (after some time) learn to direct your ch'i at animate an inanimate things.

You will soon learn that to affect living animals and people is much faster to learn. This is because you get immediate feedback from the living person or animal. Inanimate objects take longer to affect, as they have no way of communication back to you.

Ch'i is guided by your will (wei) power. Where your thoughts go so does your ch'i. You need to master yourself first. This may take some time. But if you allow yourself to practice and direct your life force around your body. For example; direct the ch'i to one hand and observe how warm and how dilated your veins will become. (Ch'i is often accompanied by dilated blood vessels. However, this is not always the case. For instance when you are startled or attacked-your body will constrict the external blood vessels and engorge the internal ones).

When you have mastered flowing ch'i from one area of your body to the next at will. Then you can start to guide the ch'i out of your body first using your hand, finger, or foot. Direct the ch'i to your arm or leg. What you are going to strive for it to project the ch'i out of your limb, just like a firearm shoots a projectile.

Unlike a firearm you will never run out of ammo. Indeed, your power is limitless. The only limit would be your lack of will-power or desire.

You must do standing ch'i kung exercise combined with deep breathing and concentration. This part can take anywhere from 3-6 months. You should experience a new world, as in new awareness of both your surroundings and your body.

Allow your mind to flow freely as you concentrate on just our breathing and guide your ch'i deep into your bones and then into your muscles.

The stance you should use is "Ma-bo" or horse riding stance stand with your feet a bit wider than shoulder width an squat down slightly. Now with your mouth closed touch the roof of your mouth with your tongue (just behind your front teeth), contract your anal sphincter as you tuck your tail bone slightly forward and down. Now both palms should be held horizontal to the ground or floor shoulders should be wide an flex and contract your back muscles several times. Creating a huge muscular triangle of flesh which is your back muscles working in synergy combined with ch'i and breath control.

The tongue touching on the roof of your mouth and the contracted anal sphincter complete the closed circuit of ch'i. This has often been called the 'micro-cosmic orbit'. In time you can imagine your body as a glass sculpture inside is a gas (ch'i) you will the gas to travel from top to bottom of your body, faster and faster. As each time you do this your ch'i will increase in power.

While I was in South Korea, my Tae Kwon Do intructor, in our 'dojang'. Should me some advanced exercises before I left the country. He said; "If you do these daily you will never get sick and always remain healthy."

He called these exercises; Ki Gong is a system of Korean exercises that stimulate and develop the mind, body and spirit. Ki, pronounced "key", is the energy that flows through your body. Ki Gong is the method used to balance the energy in your body to improve your own health and well-being.

Ki Gong will benefit you by improving your circulatory system, stimulating your immune system, and strengthening your internal organs.

Ki Gong has been known to increase flexibility, metabolism and blood circulation; improve balance, muscle and respiratory control; reduce stress; and increase blood oxidation. Ki Gong is a gentle form of exercise that can be beneficial from a standing or sitting position.

So, even though China and Korea are separated and Japan even more so. They all share the sam 'core' about mastering this mysterious life energy- Ch'i.

Ancient wood-block print demonstrating Ch'i Kung.

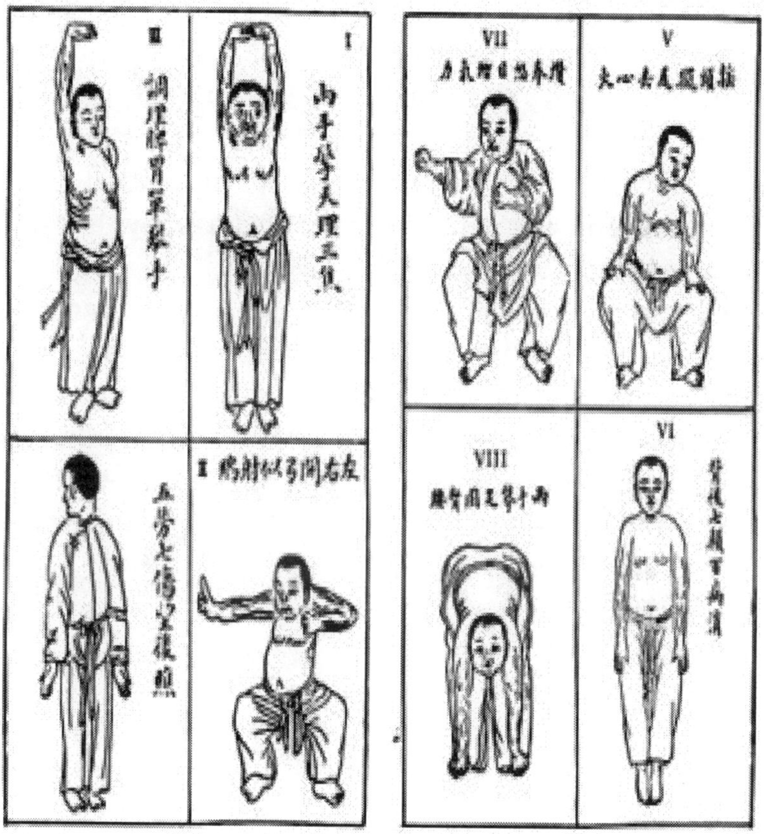

Now this alone is a good exercise to do. You may never go beyond that as so many people who practice Tai Ch'i Chuan. It is said; "The number of people who practice Tai Ch'i Chuan are like the number of hairs on the back of a bull. The number of people who achieve immortality practicing Tai Ch'i Chuan are like the horns of the bull."

This can be achieved by anyone who practices and does the exercises on a daily basis. Moving the ch'i inside your own body is a fact and it is the basic manipulation of ch'i by acupressure and acupuncture inside your body that can heal you in this way.

The next step is to make breathing deeply second nature to you and keep the ch'i flowing fast and then be able to release it towards a target or opponent. (It is here that people lose faith in this advanced form of exercise by projecting the ch'i outside of your own body at targets or from the chakras in the palms of your hands called 'lao kun' to heal people. This is also known as 'laying on of palms'.

Longevity and legends

Li Ching-Yuen was born in 1677 in Qijiang County, Sichuan province. According to a 1930 New York Times article, Professor Wu Chung-chieh of the Chengdu University discovered Imperial Chinese government records from 1827, congratulating Li Ching-Yuen on his 150th birthday, and further documents later congratulating him on his 200th birthday in 1877. In 1928, a New York Times correspondent wrote that many of the old men in Li's neighborhood asserted that their grandfathers knew him when they were boys, and that he at that time was a grown man. His obituary in the New York Times reiterates these claims. He began gathering herbs in the mountain ranges at the age of ten, and also began learning of longevity methods, surviving on a diet of herbs and rice wine (and he did eat a large bowl of cooked meat made from chicken, pig, and goat-very high protein). He lived this way for the first 40 years of his life and was very tall standing between 6' 3" and 6' 5". In 1749, when he was 71 years old, he moved to Kai Xian to join the Chinese army as a teacher of the martial arts and as an advisor.

One of his disciples, the Taijiquan Master Da Liu told of Master Li's story: at 130 years old Master Li encountered an older hermit, over 500 years old, in the mountains who taught him Baguazhang (one of three main internal martial arts the other two are Tai Ch'i Chuan, and Hsing-i-Chuan) and a set of Ch'i kung with breathing instructions, movements training coordinated with specific sounds, and dietary recommendations. Baguazhang is a soft and internal martial arts style. By internal, it is meant that early training focuses on the mind and understanding the interplay between what is being done both on the inside (mind) and outside (movements). Eventually this translates to external uses. In other words, the actual movements and techniques.

Baguazhang is often characterized by slow moving, flowing forms. That said, there are differences between the various styles.

The main purpose of Baguazhang is to improve health. It is about the flow between the mind and body. The theory behind learning this art form is that once it is understood, a person's overall life and balance will improve. Meditation and using one's energy effectively are a part of it all.

As a martial arts style, Baguazhang teaches practitioners how to use an opponent's own aggressiveness or energy against them. It is not a hard style. In other words, power on power moves are not emphasized.

Da Liu reports that his master said that his longevity "is due to the fact that I performed the exercises every day – regularly, correctly, and with sincerity – for 120 years." Returning home, he died a year later, some say of natural causes; others claim that he told friends that "I have done all I have to do in this world. I will now go home." After Li's death,

General Yang Sen investigated the truth about his claimed background and age and wrote a report about his findings that was later published.

He worked as a herbalist, selling lingzhi, goji berry, wild ginseng, he shou wu and gotu kola along with other Chinese herbs, and lived off a diet of these herbs and rice wine. Li had also supposedly produced over 200 descendants during his life span, surviving 23 wives!

While this legendary master was indeed old. It may be that his youngest son (which could have carried his name). Continued on living and being in the mountains as his father (the original Li Chen-Yuen) did. If his father lived to the age of 110-120 years old. He son (or one of them) could have lived an equally long life. The resulting error would have combined his age with his fathers making him an easy over the age of 200 years. This is just a theory, but a plausible one.

The other more staggering possibility, is that he was over 200 years old and actually at one time encountered a much older Taoist in the mountains that was an incredible 500 years old!

While I was in China, I had the pleasure of meeting and training with two very old Tai Ch'i Chuan masters. They did not look older than say an average 60-70 year old.

However, when I finally found out how old the both were (one was 101 and the other a spry 103 years old respectively) I ask them what was different that they did to look and be so much younger looking and remain in good health.

My friend translated this for me as follows: "We both have out lived our wives and a third of our children. We have only one secret if you could call it that, Tai Ch'i, Tai, Ch'i, Tai Ch'i. Everyday we both come down to this park from our apartment (which was on the 9th floor and they used the stairs) and practiced Tai Ch'i Chuan before every meal".

The key is indeed to keep active and not stagnant. What exercise that keeps you inhaling deeply, and circulating the blood, combined with stretching and deep mental concentration is an excellent way to keep in good health and also enjoy life.

Glossary of Chinese herb's and more

The following 50 herb's are the ones used in traditional Chinese medicine. After these 50 herb's I have included many more herbs because of the benefit that they can provide for all people that may have slight to harsh health problems.

Botanical name—Chinese name—English name
Agastache rugosa—huò xiang —Korean Mint
Alangium chinense—ba jiao feng—Chinese Alangium Root
Anemone chinensis—bái tóu weng—Chinese anemone
Anisodus tanguticus —shan làng dàng—Marlberry
Aster tataricus—zi wan—Tartar aster
Astragalus propinquus—huáng qí—Chinese astragalus
Camellia sinensis—chá shù—Tea Plant
Cannabis sativa—dà má—Cannabis
Carthamus tinctorius—hóng hua— Safflower
Cinnamomum cassia—ròu gùi—Chinese Cinnamon
Cissampelos pareira—xí sheng téng —Velvet leaf
Coptis chinensis—duan è huáng lián— Chinese Goldthread
Corydalis ambigua—yán hú suo—Fumewort
Croton tiglium—ba dòu —Purging Croton
Daphne—genkwa yuán hua—Lilac Daphne
Datura metel—yáng jin hua—Devil's Trumpet
Datura stramonium—zi hua màn tuó luó —Jimson Weed
Dendrobium nobile—shí hú—Noble Dendrobium
Dichroa febrifuga—cháng shan—Chinese Quinine

Botanical name—Chinese name—English name
Ephedra sinica—cao má huáng—Chinese ephedra
Eucommia ulmoides—dù zhòng —Hardy rubber tree
Euphorbia pekinensis—dà ji —Peking spurge
Flueggea suffruticosa— yi yè —Weeping Forsythia
Gentiana loureiroi—dì ding —Chinese Honeylocust
Glycyrrhiza uralensis—gan cao — Licorice
Hydnocarpus anthelminticus—dà feng zi—Chaulmoogra tree
Ilex purpurea—dongqing—Purple Holly
Leonurus japonicus—yì mu cao—Chinese motherwort
Ligusticum wallichii—chuan xiong —Szechwan lovage
Lobelia chinensis—bàn bian lián—Creeping Lobelia
Phellodendron amurense—huáng bai—Amur cork tree
Platycladus orientalis—cè bai—Chinese Arborvitae
Pseudolarix amabilis—jin qián song—Golden Larch
Psilopeganum sinense—shan má huáng— Naked rue
Pueraria lobata—gé gen—Kudzu
Rauwolfia serpentina shégenmù— cóng shégenmù— Indian Snakeroot.
Rehmannia glutinosa—gan dìhuáng—Chinese Foxglove
Rheum officinale—yào yòng dà huáng—Chinese rhubarb
Rhododendron—tsinghaiense Qing hai dù juan— ?
Saussurea costus—yún mù xiang—Costus root
Schisandra chinensis—wu wèi zi—Chinese Magnolia Vine
Scutellaria baicalensis—huáng qín—Baikal Skullcap
Stemona tuberos—bai bù — ?
Stephania tetrandra—fáng ji—Stephania Root
Styphnolobium japonicum—huái— Pagoda Tree

Botanical name—Chinese name—English name
Trichosanthes —kirilowii gua lóu—Chinese Cucumber
Wikstroemia indica —liao ge wáng —Indian stringbush

Herb's for minor to major health conditions

Acacia , Gum Arabic, Cassie flower, Catechu, Egyptian thorn
Botanical Name
Acacia senegal

The Egyptians used acacia as a fixative for ink, and to coat the bandages of most mummy's, and the gum is mentioned frequently in ancient Egyptian inscriptions. Acacia was used by the Egyptian, and pre-Egyptian healers in medicinal preparations for its soothing properties on inflamed mucus membranes, and to treat coughs and catarrh. Theophrastus, in the third and fourth centuries before Christ, described it, as also did Dioscorides and Pliny, under the name "Egyptian Gum."

Acacia has been connected to a reverence for the dead, resurrection and immortality in many religious traditions and magical contexts. Egyptians burned acacia wreaths to honor the dead, and Hebrews planted the trees to mark graves. In Voodun and African-American conjure acacia in used with Frankincense and Myrrh in rituals to contact the dead and to open the mind to visions. Catherine Yronwode Hoodoo Herb and Root Magic: A Materia Magica of African-American Conjure, and Traditional Formulary.

Acacia has the mournful distinction of supplying the crown of thorns at Golgatha. Various other plants have been named in different countries, the hawthorn, barberry and holly among them, but in the Near East, where the legend arose, only the acacia was considered to be the provider of the spiny crown.

Acai Berry , Acai Berry, jussara, Açaí
Botanical Name
Euterpe oleracea
Acai was first used by tribes in the Amazon for various medicinal purposes, among them the ability to build and strengthen the immune system, fight infection, protect the heart, and as a natural remedy for erectile dysfunction. It was also revered as an energy food, and was traditionally pulped to make wine. Mountain Rose Herbs
The genus is named after the muse Euterpe of Greek mythology.

Calamus root , Sweet Sledge. Sweet Myrtle, Sweet Flag
Botanical Name
Acorus calamus
In traditional Chinese medicine sweet flag is used to treat deafness, dizziness and epilepsy. It is used by the Akha people of Thailand for stomachache. The Chinese use it for vomiting, diarrhea, abdominal pain, and dysentery.
Calamus Side Effects: The essential oil of calamus contains aserone, which has a high toxicity. In high doses, it is

hallucinogenic. European varieties have a low concentration of aserone compared to those from India. The FDA has issued warnings about the marketing of Aserone contained in Calamus extract as a "Legal Ecstasy", and does not permit the use of calamus in food products. Do not use this herb internally without the supervision of a qualified expert. Use the whole herb only in external applications; never use the essential oil of calamus in extract form.

Agaricus blazei mushroom , Himematsutake, (Japan) Cogumelo do Sol (Brazil)
Botanical Name
Agaricus blazei
Agaricus blazei is one of the most popular medicinal and culinary mushrooms with a delicious almond extract flavor and meaty texture. This species of mushroom native to Brazil, and widely cultivated in Japan for its medicinal uses. A. blazei has been used in complementary and alternative medicine to treat many immune disorders and is being studied as a treatment for cancer. It was traditionally used to treat many common diseases like cardiovascular disease, hepatitis, high blood cholesterol, diabetes, and skin disorders like eczema.

Agave syrup , Agave nectar, Agave syrup
Botanical Name
Agave tequilana,
Increasing evidence now suggests that the rise in

consumption of carbohydrates, particularly refined sugars high in fructose, are a very important contributing factor in the development of obesity and type 2 diabetes. Agave is used as a healthier alternative to refined sugars in part because of it's low glycemic index which helps to prevent spikes in blood sugar. Is agave a good alternative for diabetics? The answer, sadly may be no. Agave is certainly a great improvement over HFS and cane sugar, however Agave nectar typically is primarily fructose, which can still cause problems for diabetics if consumed without care.

Agrimony , Liverwort, cockleburr, sticklewort
Botanical Name
Agrimonia eupatoria L.
In traditional Chinese medicine In traditional Chinese medicine, agrimony is a major herb for stopping bleeding and it is used to treat profuse menstruation. Chinese research indicates that agrimony can increase coagulation of the blood.

Ajwain Seed , Ajwan, Ajwon
Botanical Name
Trachyspermum ammi
Syn. Carum copticum
Ajwain is very similar to its western relatives in the plant family Apiaceae Cumin, Dill and Parsley, both in the way it is used in food and in medicine. The high concentration of essential oils in ajwain seeds, primarily thymol, give them an aroma and

flavor resembling thyme, with a stronger bite. Ajwain seeds are used to flavor vegetables and fish in Indian cuisine and are fried in oil or ghee(clarified butter) to mellow the acrid taste.

Alder Buckthorn , Alder Dogwood, Alder Buckthorn
Botanical Name
Rhamnus frangula
Syn. Frangula alnus
The dried and aged bark is the part used in herbal medicine, primarily as a laxative. Frangula bark is considered to be milder in action than aloes and senna with only minimal irritant properties, about the same as rhubarb. It is a close relative of the California buckthorn, Cascara sagrada The slightly gentler action makes it more suitable to those with chronic constipation as a tonic to re-educate the bowel. For persistent cases frangula with not suffice on its own and is often combined with carminatives and stronger laxatives.

Alfalfa
Botanical Name
Medicago sativa L.
In traditional Chinese medicine Alfalfa known as Mu-Su in Chinese medicine, made its way to China during the late Han Dynasty(around 2000 A.D.) from Persia. One of its most common uses in Chinese medicine is in the treatment of ulcers. It is also used to strengthen digestion and stimulate appetite ,plus it contains the most minerals besides kelp.

Allspice , Pimento, Jamaica Pepper
Botanical Name
Pimenta officinalis
Allspice, Pimenta officinalis , is an aromatic, digestive stimulant, whose taste, aroma and properties resemble a combination of cloves, juniper berries, cinnamon, and pepper. The essential oil extracted from allspice contains a good deal of eugenol, the same oil extracted from cloves. Adding allspice to herbal teas as well as foods aids in digestion.

Almond Oil
Botanical Name
Prunus dulcis
Sweet almond oil is a favorite in aroma-therapy as a carrier oil and is valued in natural skin care for it's ability to soften and condition the skin. Pale yellow in color, almond oil is expelled pressed from raw almond kernels. The oil contains glucosides, minerals and vitamins and is rich in protein. Almond oil is good for all skin types and helps to relieve dryness, itching and inflammation.

Almonds are a rich source of Vitamin E, and mono unsaturated fat, one of the two "good" fats responsible for lowering LDL cholesterol. Almond nuts are a healthy treat as is, or can be made into almond butter, a spread similar to peanut butter. The sweet almond contains practically no carbohydrates and can be made into flour for those on a low carbohydrate diet, suffering from diabetes, or by those who are looking for a gluten free flour.

Aloe Vera Gel
Botanical Name
Aloe vera
Syn. Aloe barbadensis
Aloe gel skin care: Aloe vera gel is an indispensable part of your herbal dispensary. The leaf juices of the aloe plant have important medicinal uses making aloe one of the most respected medicinal plants found in many gels, creams and lotions. Modern researchers have identified several reasons why aloe gel spurs wound healing: It has antibacterial, antifungal and antiviral compounds that help prevent wound infections. It also has immune-stimulating and anti-inflammatory compounds, and it stimulates collagen synthesis and skin regeneration after a burn. Aloe gel contains vitamins C and E, plus the mineral zinc. Aloe vera gel is soothing, anti-inflammatory, and antibacterial - helps heal acne, improve the appearance of wrinkles, and hydrate damaged skin. Applying a thin layer of aloe vera gel will help ease discomfort caused by painful skin irritations, and acne.

Amalaki, amla , Indian gooseberry, aamla, amalika
Botanical Name
Phyllanthus emblica
Syn. Emblica officinalis
Amalaki is one of three fruits used in the Ayurvedic herbal

formula called triphala (which, in Hindi/Sanskrit, means literally "three fruits"). 1These fruits in combination are thought to balance the three doshas : Amalaki is sour and balances pitta. Bibhitaki (Terminalia belerica) is sweet and pungent and balances kapha, and haritaki (Terminalia chebula) is bitter and balances vata. This formula is used to treat obesity, and can be especially effective and safe for chronic constipation.

Ginseng Root, American
Botanical Name
Panax quinquefolius
In Chinese traditions, American ginseng is considered to be more yin, helping to reduce the heat of the respiratory and digestive systems.

Angelica root , Choraka
Botanical Name
Angelica archangelica
It is closely related to Dong Quai, one of the most respected female tonics in traditional Chinese medicine. Angelica is a traditional birthing herb used to help bring on a delayed labor and to help expel the placenta following childbirth. Angelica relieves painful and cramping menstruation, (Dysmenorrhea), and brings on delayed menstruation. Angelica is especially good when bloating or cramps are present.

Anise Seed , Aniseed
Botanical Name
Pimpinella anisum
Star anise is found in many traditional Chinese and Japanese recipes for food and medicine. It is used for similar purposes as sweet anise, but is considered to be drying and warming.
Anise Seed Side Effects: Narcotic in large doses. Anise seeds contain anethole, a plant hormone similar to human estrogen, that promotes menstruation, and lactation in nursing mothers. Anise should not be used while pregnant and in young babies. The essential oil is for topical use only.

Apple , Apple cider vinegar, wine vinegar
Botanical Name
Malus domestica
Syn. M.sylvestris
The old folks really knew a good thing when they saw it. "An apple a day keeps the doctor away"; this humble fruit can help prevent two of the major lifestyle diseases of modern life, diabetes and heart disease. Apples contain malic and tartaric acids, and salts of potassium, sodium, magnesium, and iron. They also contain soluble fiber, which can lower cholesterol, help prevent plaque buildup in your arteries, and slow the uptake of glucose, helping you maintain healthy blood sugar levels.
Herbalists consider apples to be cleansing and tonic to the liver and kidneys. The best of the medicinal compounds are

contained in the apple peel.

Vinegar made from apples, was considered a medicine by the Egyptians, Romans and prescribed by Hippocrates (Greece) for internal and external protection against many diseases. Caesar's armies used vinegar as a beverage, Helen of Troy bathed in it to relax. During the First World War medics used vinegar to treat soldiers' wounds.

Argemone - Prickly Poppy , Mexican Poppy, bluestem
Botanical Name
Argemone mexicana
Syn. A. albiflora
This plant is very popular among those seeking a "legal high" and the mildly narcotic seeds are often mixed with tobacco or other herbs in smoking mixtures. However, most content themselves to growing the plant for its attractive flowers in native habitat gardens. Like other members of the poppy family, the prickly poppy has a long history as a traditional medicine.

Arjuna
Botanical Name
Terminalia arjuna
Arjuna is among the most frequently prescribed herbs for cardiovascular health in ayurvedic medicine. Modern studies confirm its beneficial effects on managing lipid levels and hypertension.1 The bark of the arjuna tree contains calcium

salts, magnesium salts, tannins, and saponin glycosides which may be the primary source for arjuna's beneficial effects on the heart. Other traditional uses include : hemorrhages, diarrhea, dysentery, edema, skin problems, and fractures. In addition, it has been found to have antibacterial and anti-mutagenic properties.

Artichoke, Globe
Botanical Name
Cynara scolymus
Medicinal Uses of Artichoke leaves Teas and extracts made from the leaves of the artichoke plant are a traditional tonic for the liver and gallbladder. Both laboratory and clinical studies strongly suggest artichoke leaf extract to be a good therapeutic option in dyspeptic syndrome. (irritable stomach, nervous gastropathy, flatulence, irritable colon, functional biliary tract disease).

Asafoetida root , devil's dung, food of the gods, hing, narthex
Botanical Name
Ferula asafoetida
Asafoetida is useful as a digestive spice that has the additional benefit of lowering cholesterol and reducing gas. The pungent oil can be using to repel insects. Asafoetida was one of the most commonly prescribed herbs in the 19th century in the treatment of hysteria and for many symptoms associated with mood swings and depression, or in ayurvedic terms "Asafetida

is a grounding herb that can therefore balance an overactive, over emotional, turbulent system".

Ashwagandha root , Ashwaganda, Ajagandha, Indian ginseng, Winter cherry
Botanical Name
Withania somnifera
Ashwagandha is often touted as the Indian version of ginseng because, like ginseng, ashwagandha is revered as a non-specific tonic and adaptogen. Adaptogens are important in cases of ongoing, chronic stress. Ashwagandha root rejuvenates without being over stimulating, so is more useful than ginseng in weakened and debilitated persons.

Asparagus , Satavari
Botanical Name
Asparagus spp
There are over 300 species in the asparagus family, many are used medicinally, grown as ornaments or eaten as vegetables. The most well-known species, Asparagus officinalis, is what we commonly refer to as asparagus, whose tasty green stalks are one the most nutritious of the early green vegetables in the spring garden. Like tomatoes, it is high is lycopene, a powerful antioxidant that is protective against many degenerative diseases and cancers. The vitamin A content is important for eye health and the fibrous stalks help to reduce cholesterol. Asparagus is also a useful diuretic and mild laxative.

Astragalus root , Huang qi , yellow leader
Botanical Name
astragalus membranaceus
Syn. A. propinquus

In traditional Chinese medicine The Chinese knowledge of the astragalus is much older than here in the West dating back at least 2,000 years. In traditional Chinese medicine, astragalus is one of the 50 fundamental herbs and is used in numerous Chinese prescriptions in fu-zheng therapy. Fu-zheng refers to treating disease by either enhancing or promoting the defense mechanism or normalizing the central energy. It is considered sweet and mildly warm, tonifying of the qi.

Avocado
Botanical Name
Persea americana

Avocados are a favorite food because of the high fat content that gives them such a creamy, luscious flavor. This puts some dieters off, it shouldn't. Most of the fat contained in avocados is mono-unsaturated fat, about 75 percent in a typical avocado. The fruit also has more potassium than bananas and is rich in B vitamins, Vitamin E and Vitamin K. There are some recent studies that confirm avocados role in maintaining healthy cholesterol levels, adding to the long list of reasons to enjoy this luscious, medicinal food.

Bacopa , Water hyssop, Brahmi
Botanical Name
Bacopa monnieri
Bacopa appears to strengthen memory and improve concentration by enhancing the conductivity of nerve tissue. It is relatively new here in the West, and has garnered a good deal of buzz as a nootropic supplement used to enhance memory, but has been used in traditional Ayurvedic medicine since ancient times to treat mental illness and a range of mental functions. Traditional applications and in vitro lab studies show that Bacopa has a direct effect on improving brain functions, increasing concentration, and in promoting memory functions.

Barberry , Huang Lian, Chinese Goldthread, Pepperidge-bush, Daru Haridra
Botanical Name
Berberis vulgaris L.
Both Chinese goldthread (native to the mountains of Szechwan province in China) and the barberry known in Europe and North America are rich natural sources of berberine.

Basil , Sweet Basil
Botanical Name
Ocimum basilicum
Basil is one of the best loved culinary herbs for good reason. Basil improves appetite and like other herbs in the mint family

it settles the stomach, improves appetite and is a natural disinfectant. Basil is known for its many varieties, many with distinct aromas that come from different qualities in their essential oils contained in the leaves. The strong clove scent of sweet basil comes from eugenol, the citrus scent of lemon basil and lime basil comes from a higher portion of the aldehyde citral and limonene, which gives actual lemon peel its scent. African blue basil has a strong camphor smell because it has camphor and camphene in higher proportions. Anise basil contains anethole, the same chemical that makes anise smell like licorice, and in fact is sometimes called anise basil.

White Kidney Bean
Botanical Name
Phaseolus vulgaris
Spikes in blood sugar and increased insulin levels begins the progression to insulin insensitivity and type 2 diabetes. Common staples in the American diet, white bread, rice and potatoes consist of monosaccharides which are absorbed quickly in the intestine. These "high glycemic foods" can also be key factors in the development of cardiovascular disease and obesity. Many studies have shown that Phaseolus vulgaris, the common white bean is an inhibitor of alpha-amylase, an enzyme that promotes the breakdown of starch in the human gastrointestinal tract. Ingestion of this inhibitor helps prevent the breakdown of the carbohydrate in the intestine in foods so

the less sugars are absorbed as fat cells for future use. Raspberries (Rubus idaeus ssp. idaeus) and strawberries (Fragaria spp.) contain anthocyanins which inhibit a-amylase activity and ellagitannins and have shown similar effects. The most amount of research along these lines has been done on white beans.

Uva Ursi , Bearberry

Botanical Name

Arctostaphylos uva-ursi

Uva ursi contains a considerable amount of tannins (up to 40 percent) making it one of natures most powerful astringents. Unlike most herbs which can have a wide range of uses, uva-ursi is a specialist in infections and inflammations of the urniary tract. Uva uris ontains as assortment of chemical compounds, especially arbutin, that are active against many of the pathogens commonly found in urinary tract infections.

Bilberry , Huckleberry

Botanical Name

Vaccinium myrtillus

Bilberry has beneficial effects on many disorders from poor vision and diabetes to high cholesterol and blood pressure. Because capillary damage is the primary factor in a number of eye diseases, such as diabetic retinopathy, glaucoma, and cataracts, bilberry extracts are often promoted as a source of protection. This great tasting berry also finds a place in the home herbalist's medicine cabinet as a simple and effective remedy for reducing bruises from ‘black eyes’.

Bitter Melon , balsam pear, bitter gourd, Karela
Botanical Name
Momordica charantia
The gourd-like fruit has a long history in Chinese and Ayurvedic Medicine both a healthy food and medicine and its use as a treatment for diabetes is supported by scientific studies here in the west. Bitter melon improves the body's ability to use blood sugar and improves glucose tolerances. James Duke writes "One of the phytochemicals, charantin is said to be more potent than tolbutamide, and has fewer side effects." and recommends eating one small melon a day 1 Several clinical trials have shown that bitter melon extract and juice lower blood sugar in people with type 1 or type 2 diabetes. There is good scientific evidence that bitter melon is effective at reducing blood glucose levels in diabetics.

Black Cohosh root , Black snake root, Squaw Root, Bugbane
Botanical Name
Cimicifuga racemosa
Syn. Actaea racemosa
Black cohosh contains numerous chemical constituents, among them isoflavones which mimic hormonal activity. This makes this herb useful for hot flashes, vaginal dryness, and even the depression sometimes associated with menopause.

Though black and blue cohosh are unrelated botanically they are often used together in formulas to support the female reproductive system. Blue cohosh acts primarily as a uterine stimulant, while black cohosh effects estrogen levels

Black Pepper
Botanical Name
Piper nigrum
Pepper is one of the oldest known spices, and was important enough to early medicine to be included in the Herbals of Dioscorides and Galen. The uses of black pepper go far beyond the kitchen where pepper stimulates the taste buds. Black pepper is stimulating to the digestive system, expectorates coughs, and helps to clear the lungs of congestion. Black pepper is added to turmeric and many other herbal formulations as an activator.

Black Seed oil , Kalonjii, Black cumin, black caraway, Roman-coriander, fennel-flower
Botanical Name
Nigella sativa
Black seed, sometimes called nigella seed, is used in both whole seed and seed oil form as a healthy dietary supplement. Black seed contains fatty acids, vitamins and minerals in a unique cell structure. Native to Western Asia, Turkey, Iraq, and Egypt, black seed oil has been valued for it's health benefits for centuries. It is said that Cleopatra used black seed oil to

keep her hair soft and shiny.

Black Walnut
Botanical Name
Juglans nigra
Walnuts are a good source dietary source of serotonin, which is important in maintaining a healthy emotional balance. A lack of serotonin in the brain is thought to be a cause of depression.
Walnuts are also one of the best plant based sources of omega-3 fatty acids. Both research and population studies have shown that having the right balance of omega-3 fatty acids in the diet reduces inflammation and may help lower risk such as heart disease, cancer, and auto-immune disorders such as rheumatoid arthritis.

Raspberry Leaf , Raspberry Leaf
Botanical Name
Rubus idaeus
The fruit is rich in nutrients and helps to combat anaemia. In Chinese medicine, Chinese raspberries (the fruit) are used to strengthen the kidneys and to treat enuresis.
The wild tangle of thorny trailing vines yield a tasty fruit, but it is the leaves that are of interest to the herbalist. Raspberry leaf is a mild and safe medicinal food, and the toothy leaves are commonly used to treat diarrhea, colds, and stomach complaints. An effective and safe remedy for children,

raspberry tea is given to reduce fever and calm diarrhea. Raspberry is good tonic herb with a rich supply of vitamins and minerals that help build strong bones and general good health. It can be taken long term and is generally considered safe with no unwanted side effects.

Kelp/Bladderwrack , Fucus, Seaweed, dried
Botanical Name
Fucus vesiculosis
Kelp, dried seaweed Fucus vesiculosis, was the original source of iodine, which does not occur in nature in the uncombined condition but is widely, though sparingly, distributed in the form of iodides and iodates, chiefly of sodium and potassium, in seawater, some seaweeds, and various mineral and medicinal springs. Kelp is an important part of the diet in Japan, Norway, and Scotland. For vegans (vegetarians who eat no animal products at all), it supplies vitamin B12, otherwise found almost exclusively in animal products, and is a concentrated source of minerals, including iodine, potassium, magnesium, calcium, and iron. As a source of iodine, it assists in the production of of thyroid hormones, which are necessary for maintaining healthy metabolism in all cells of the body. The brown algae known as bladderwrack is a particularly common source of kelp.

Blessed Thistle , Holy thistle, St. Benedict's thistle
Botanical Name
Cnicus benedictus
Syn. Carbenia benedicta
Blessed thistle is a bitter tonic, and as such is an excellent digestive herb to use as an apertif to prevent gas and bloating from eating a meal heavy in fats. Blessed thistle herb is also considered a depurative, having diuretic and diaphoretic properties; these actions help to purify the system and rid the body of toxins. Blessed thistle's medicinal actions help give support to the liver and help it to repair itself.
There is supporting research to suggest that blessed thistle has anti-tumor and anticancer effects. This adds another reason for those who are at risk for cancer to consider the use of blessed thistle as a tonic herb.
Blessed thistle is a traditional tonic for women. Dong quai and wild yam, along with other estrogenic herbs can be used in combination with blessed thistle to treat menstrual difficulties and other conditions where a woman's hormones need to be brought back into balance.

Bloodroot , red puccoon blood root, pauson
Botanical Name
Sanguinaria canadensis L
Bloodroot's name is derived from the color of the reddish roots which contain the phytochemical sanguinarine- The red juice from the root is used externally in pastes and salves to remove

warts, skin tags, and some skin cancers. Eclectic doctors in the late 1800's formulated "black" salves with bloodroot, flour, water, and zinc chloride and applied it directly to tumors and other cancers. Blood root does have the unique ability to dissolve abnormal skin growths, however skin cancers should not be self-treated, it is especially important not to try to remove a blue or black skin tumor with blood root. These could be melanoma, and must be treated by a physician.

Blue Cohosh Root , squaw root
Botanical Name
Caulophyllum thalictroides
Blue cohosh is considered to be one of the best herbs to bring on menstruation, and is one of the traditional herbs used to induce labor in natural childbirth. It contains the phytochemical calulopsponin which actively stimulates uterine contractions and promotes blood flow to the pelvic region. 1 Blue cohosh is generally used in combination with other herbs, often black cohosh, to treat menstrual disorders. The herb's powerful antispasmodic properties are helpful in relieving the menstrual cramps of a painful period.

Vervain , Blue Vervain, Wild Hyssop, Simpler's Joy, Herb of the cross
Botanical Name
Verbena hastata, V. officinalis
Vervain has been useful to herbal healers for many centuries

of recorded history, both in the Europe (Verbena officinalis)Netje Blanchan and in North America, (V. hastata),yet there is a dearth of human studies with this herb. Vervain's healing properties are attributed primarily to its bitter and stimulating effect on the liver and other organs, as well as its relaxing effect on the nervous system. Vervain is useful in many diseases as a pain reliever and natural tranquilizer, an expectorant used to treat chronic bronchitis, and an antirheumatic used to relive joint pain. Herbalists consider vervain especially helpful when depression is related to chronic illness. As an added benefit, it can help to heal any damage that has occurred to the liver.

Blueberries , blueberry, huckleberry, ligonberry
Botanical Name
Vaccinium spp
Syn. Vaccinium corymbosum
Blueberries are a naturally delicious treat that can be enjoyed without hesitation - a totally guilt free pleasure. There are many different species of North American blueberries adapted to thrive in climates from Alaska (Vaccinium alaskaense) to the Carolina farkleberry (Vaccinium arboreum). Blueberries are of special interest in the functional/medicinal food category due to the high levels of anthocyanin and polyphenolic antioxidant compounds they contain. Blueberries have a higher antioxidant capacity (in some cases as high as 40-50 mmoles TE/g) than other healthy fruits and vegetables.

Bogbean , Buckbean, March Clover
Botanical Name
Menyanthes trifoliata
Bogbean is one of the medicinal plants that containing iridoids, plant chemicals that play a central role in herbalism as they are often the basis of what is known as the bitter principle. These bitter tonics, such as bogbean stimulate digestive secretions, including bile.

Boldo
Botanical Name
Peumus boldus Molina
The use of boldo is passed down from the time of the Incas and the herb is used in much the same way today - for a wide range of stomach, digestive, and liver complaints. Boldo leaves are used to treat bladder and urinary tract infections, gallbladder discomfort, gallstones, heartburn and indigestion, and stomach cramps. The herb works by encouraging the release of bile and dissolving fats and also by increasing intestinal transit time, giving the digestive tract more time to digest food. The ascaridole in boldo attacks intestinal worms.

Boneset , Common Thorough wort, Agueweed, Indian Sage
Botanical Name
Eupatorium perfoliatum
This Native American remedy for colds and fever was adopted by early settlers to America. The name refers to the plant's use

to treat breakbone fever, (dengue), a viral infection that causes such intense muscle pain that sufferers feel their bones will break. Only the advent of aspirin displaced boneset as the popular choice for home remedies. Boneset is still one of the best herbal remedies for the flu and fevers.

Borage Seed Oil
Botanical Name
Borago officinalis
Borage seed oil has the highest concentration of gamma linolenic acid (GLA) naturally found, higher than in any other plant source. Borage can be used as a supplement to correct EFA deficiencies in chronic inflammatory conditions, most notably rheumatoid arthritis. Borage oil is also good choice for skin disorders such as psoriasis and eczema. The high content of essential fatty acids in borage oil as well as its depurative nature make it a great skin conditioner that re-hydrates and revitalizes sun damaged or aged skin.

Boswellia (Frankincense) , Olibanum, Indian Frankincense, Arabic Frankincense, and Salai guggal
Botanical Name
Boswellia thurifera
Supplements containing boswellic acids combined with glucosamine are often used to relieve the joint pain and reduce inflammation in all types of arthritis . Boswellia or Indian frankincense is one of the Ayurvedic gum resins which

are referred to collectively as guggals.

Pineapple
Botanical Name
Ananas comosus
Pineapple contains a proteolytic enzyme bromelain, which digests food by breaking down protein. Only modest quantities of bromelain are in the edible parts of the fruit, all commercially all commercially available bromelain is derived from the stem. Bromelain supplements are particularly popular among athletes for treating all sorts of physical aches and injuries. There are questions about how well bromelain is absorbed, and to many herbal authorities the value may be overstated. Nature gave us many similar proteolytic enzymes, (like Ginger), that are more highly concentrated in the edible parts of the plants. Pineapple is healthy fruit, a good source of manganese, as well as containing significant amounts of Vitamin C.

Buchu
Botanical Name
Agathosma betulina
Syn. Barosma betulina
The leaves of the buchu are an effective diuretic, are antimicrobial and anti-inflammatory. These medicinal properties make buchu effective in the treatment of bladder and urinary tract infections (UTI),and kidney infections, and

buchu is also often used to treat prostate infections. Buchu's healing and soothing properties indicate its use in combination with other relevant remedies for many conditions affecting the urinary tract. Buchu is often combined with couchgrass, corn silk, cranberry, cleavers, dandelion, goldenrod, parsley, and uva ursi.

Alder Buckthorn , Alder Dogwood, Alder Buckthorn
Botanical Name
Rhamnus frangula
Syn. Frangula alnus
The dried and aged bark is the part used in herbal medicine, primarily as a laxative. Frangula bark is considered to be milder in action than aloes and senna with only minimal irritant properties, about the same as rhubarb. It is a close relative of the California buckthorn, Cascara sagrada The slightly gentler action makes it more suitable to those with chronic constipation as a tonic to re-educate the bowel. For persistent cases frangula with not suffice on its own and is often combined with carminatives and stronger laxatives.

Cascara Sagrada , Buckthorn
Botanical Name
Rhamnus purshiana DC
Dried, aged cascara sagrada bark is often prescribed for chronic constipation. The herb must be allowed to age at least a year before use to break down its anthrone chemicals. The

bark contains compounds called anthraquinones (cascarosides A and B) which are transformed by intestinal bacteria into substances that act on the nerves in the intestinal tract, helping to pass stools.

Bugleweed , Water Horehound, Gypsywort
Botanical Name
Lycopus spp.
Bugleweed is a specific for overactive thyroid, especially when symptoms include shortness of breath, palpitations, and shaking. The lithospermic acid in bugleweed is believed to decrease levels of certain hormones, especially the thyroid hormone thyroxine (T3). This compound also keeps antibodies from binding to and "burning out" cells in an overactive thyroid gland. By moderating estrogen levels, bugleweed relieves cyclic breast pain in women.

Bupleurum , chai hu, Chinese thorowax root
Botanical Name
Bupleurum chinense
It's Chinese name that literally means "kindling of the barbarians." Bupleurum is a primary ingredient an ancient Chinese medicinal formula known as Xiao Chai Hu Tang, first recorded in the Treatise on Cold Induced Febrile Disease (Shang Han Lun) circa 280 AD.
Bupleurum is an important Chinese tonic herb for the liver and circulatory system that is not widely used by Western

herbalists. As with most traditional Chinese herbs, bupleurum is rarely used alone, but is often combined with ginseng, ginger, and combined with peony to treat menstrual problems, with bitter orange peel for irregularity or loss of appetite, with scutellaria for chills and fever.

Burdock root , Niu Bang Zi, Go Bo, Gobo
Botanical Name
Arctium lappa
In traditional Chinese medicine In Chinese medicine, the dried seeds are used for colds, coughs, swelling in the throat, measles and boils.
Burdock has an ancient and respected reputation as a nutritive liver tonic that helps to clean and build the blood, while its diuretic action of burdock helps in the elimination of waste materials. Taken internally, this root promotes sweating and the elimination of harmful high levels of uric acid via the kidneys. The roots, leaves, and seeds of burdock can all be used, but in commercial preparations, you'll most commonly find the root. Rich in minerals, this plant is used as a food by many cultures. Burdock helps to cleanse the body from the inside out and is most useful in those conditions that can be traced back to liver disorders or a general overload of toxins in the system including problem skin. Burdock may also play a useful role in helping to control blood sugar levels due to the inulin content of the root. In Europe, the fresh root is used for lowering blood sugar, its inulin content making it particularly

suitable for diabetes.
Burdock is very popular in Asian cuisine, both in Japan and China. The fresh root is skinned and sliced into thin rounds that are added to soups and stir-frys. Miso broth with burdock and other vegetables is a very popular soup in Japan. The young, tender leaves can be blanched and used as a salad vegetable in the spring.

Butcher's Broom , Jew's Myrtle, Sweet Broom, Scotch Broom
Botanical Name
Ruscus aculeatus
Herbalists also use this potent plant in the treatment of poor circulation, irregular heart rhythm, and other related heart problems. Broom is known for it's cleansing and diuretic properties, which makes it useful for treating bladder infections and reducing cellulite. Drinking broom root tea on a consistent basis can also help with chronic dark circles under the eyes.

Butterbur , Langwort, Umbrella Plan
Botanical Name
Petasites vulgaris
Syn. P.officinalis
What is butterbur? Butterbur root has been used traditionally since the Middle Ages, and in North America during colonial times as a heart stimulant, acting both as a cardiac tonic and also as a diuretic, to treat fevers, wheezing and colds. Modern

research supports the use of butterbur in treating the symptoms of seasonal rhinitis (allergies), and asthma. Clinical trials done with a proprietary butterbur extract, Petadolex, proved an effective therapy in the prevention of migraines.

Pleurisy Root , Butterfly-weed. Swallow-wort, Tuber root, Wind root, Colic root, Orange Milkweed
Botanical Name
Asclepias tuberosa
Pleurisy root gets its name from its medicinal uses against a wide range of respiratory and lung conditions specifically pleurisy, inflammation of the lining of the lungs and chest (the pleura) that leads to sharp pains in the chest when you take a breath or cough. It was formerly official to the United States Pharmacopoeia for pleurisy, but outside the herbal community, this herb is best known as butterfly weed for its attraction of butterflies, particularly monarchs.

Butternut , White walnut, Lemon walnut
Botanical Name
Juglans cinerea
Butternut is a close relative of the black walnut and the two are often combined in herbal preparations. Herbalists use the inner bark as a gentle laxative, that does not cause harsh cramping.

Cacao , Chocolate, cocoa

Botanical Name

Theobroma cacao L

Cacao Theobroma, "food of the gods" : Chocolate is made from the fermented, roasted and ground beans taken from the pods of the tropical cacao tree. There is plenty of accumulating good news for those of us who are chocolate lovers. Dark chocolate that contains a high percentage of cacao has been shown to have positive effects on mood, high blood pressure, and heart health, improving circulation and having no adverse effects on cholesterol.

There are over 350 known chemicals found in chocolate, including stimulants like caffeine, theobromine, phenylethylamine and anandamide. Theobromine, the alkaloid contained in the beans, resembles caffeine in its action, but its effect on the central nervous system is less powerful and does not have the sleep disturbing effects of caffeine. Research published makes a strong case that dark chocolate can be a powerful cough suppressant. The theobromine content of dark chocolate may actually be a more effective cough medicine than traditional or over-the counter cold and cough remedies.cough medicine making it a safe nighttime calmer for children.

Phenylethylamine (PEA) is partly responsible for the "high" that you get from eating chocolate. PEA facilitates the release of dopamine a naturally occurring chemical into your body. The neurotransmitter anandamide, also found in chocolate is responsible for the prolonged pleasurable sensation of the previous mentioned. This positive feeling can help support your diet goals along with cardiovascular exercise and reduced calorie intake. Whatever the reason recent studies show that adults who eat chocolate on a regular basis are actually thinner that those who don't and that modest, regular chocolate consumption might be calorie-neutral. The key to using chocolate is to learn to enjoy it without mixing it with loads of sugar. The darker the chocolate, the more health benefits (and less sugar) it contains.

Chocolate enjoys an reputation as an aphrodisiac, which may explain the tradition of chocolates and Valentines day. It's interesting to note that most researchers claim that women prefer chocolate over sex. Cocoa Butter is an aromatic solid butter pressed from the roasted seeds of the cacao tree that brings a supple, luxurious feel to dry skin.

Cajeput Oil , Weeping tea tree, weeping paperbark

Botanical Name Melaleuca leucadendron, M. leucadendra

Syn. Melaleuca minor

The key use of cajeput is to relieve stiff, aching joints caused by rheumatism. Cajeput oil is traditionally mixed with camphor as an external rub for arthritis and gout.

Cajeput is antibacterial and clears congestion making it a good inhalant oil for colds and sinus infections. The sweet scent of cajeput uplifts the spirit while it cleanses the air.

Apply the cajeput oil externally as first aid for burns, cramps, colic, earache, headache, muscle pain, and toothache. Cajeput is an astringent oil that can benefit oily skin and help clear eczema.

Calamus root , Sweet Sledge. Sweet Myrtle, Sweet Flag
Botanical Name
Acorus calamus
In Chinese medicine sweet flag is used to treat deafness, dizziness and epilepsy. It is used by the Akha people of Thailand for stomachache. The Chinese use it for vomiting, diarrhea, abdominal pain, and dysentery.

Calendula , Pot marigold
Botanical Name
Calendula officinalis
Calendula is a stunningly beautiful flower, the deep orange and yellow petals form a colorful contrast with the greenery in the herb garden. Is it little wonder that Calendula, called "Marygold", Marigold or "sunbride" in the herbals of the middle ages, was ascribed such magical powers and healing virtues? Calendula flower oil heals the skin very well and will also heal sores in the mouth as well as gums that are infected.

California Poppy , Gold Poppy
Botanical Name
Eschscholzia californica
California poppy is one of the oldest North American remedies

for stress-induced maladies including sensitivity to changes in the weather. The above ground parts and roots of this wildflower show promise in the treatment of insomnia without the side effects and dependency risks of sleep aids. Higher doses of California poppy are sedating, lower doses reduce anxiety and lower stress. The effect is far milder than that of opium, which contains a different class of alkaloids.

Camphor
Botanical Name
Cinnamomum camphora
Camphor oil has a duel action of hot and cold, which has a balancing effect on the yin and yang energies. When first applied camphor oil numbs and cools the peripheral nerve endings, then warms the painful area as it stimulates circulation to cold, stiff muscles and limbs. This analgesic effect of camphor makes it a favorite oil to be used in pain relieving massage blends for sore muscles, low back pain, and arthritic pain.

Canola oil rapeseed
Botanical Name
Brassica napus
Like soybean, canola contains both high oil content as well as high protein content. It contains about 40% oil and 23% protein compared to 20% and 40%, respectively, for soybean. Like soybean, when the oil is crushed out, it leaves a high

quality, high protein (37%) feed concentrate which is highly palatable to livestock. Commercial varieties of canola were developed from two species; Brassica napus (Argentine type) and Brassica campestris (Polish type). Both species of canola produce seed that is high in polyunsaturated fatty acids (oleic, linoleic, and linolenic).

Caralluma

Botanical Name

Caralluma fimbriata

Caralluma spp is a succulent plant native to Asia, the Mediterranean, and Africa. Caralluma is eaten as a food and has a number of traditional ethnobotanical uses that include: diabetes, leprosy, rheumatism, paralysis, joint pain, migraines, fever, malaria, and inflammation. The species C. fimbriata and C. adscendens var. fimbriata have been used in traditional Indian medicine in this manner. In addition, C. tuberculata has been used as a digestive aid and to treat diabetes. Today most interest is centered on caralluma's use as an appetite suppressant. Caralluma works in much the same way as hoodia; both hoodia and caralluma contain preganane glycosides thought to aid in weight loss. This is now available in health food stores and in a lot of current diet supplements.

Caraway Seed
Botanical Name
Carum carvi
Caraway is best known as the crunchy seeds atop dark rye bread but this familiar kitchen spice is also one of the best herbs to prevent gas and bloating. Caraway is also a good remedy for colds and congestion, it contains mild antihistamines, antimicrobial compounds that help to relax the muscles that cause coughing spasms. Caraway seeds are also used in a number of medicinal preparations for treating disorders such as rheumatism, eye infections and toothaches. Caraway seed oil is used in treating fungus infections as well, and is effective against candida infections. Caraway is often used in combination with peppermint oil to relieve the symptoms of irritable bowel syndrome and indigestion.

Carob , Locust Bean, St. John's-Bread
Botanical Name
Ceratonia siliqua
Carob is a healthy substitute for chocolate that is lower in calories. Roasted carob is naturally sweeter, (or not as bitter), as unsweetened chocolate, so it can be made palatable with less added sugar in recipes. Carob has a number of advantages over chocolate: it is hypo-allergenic, and hypo-glycemic. The true trick to enjoying carob is to not expect it to taste exactly like chocolate,(and be forever disappointed), but to learn to appreciate carob for its own unique taste. Which

has a slightly nutty taste combined with a unique sweetness.

Cashew Nut , Cajueiro, jambu
Botanical Name
Anacardium occidentale
Cashew nuts could possibly hold answers in the search for better ways to treat diabetes and high blood sugar. Animal studies with diabetic rats fed nut milk extract are promising, but more study is needed. Anacardium have long been used in the folk medicine and traditional cuisines of India, South America and the Caribbean. Cajueiro, as the tree is known in Brazil contains naturally occurring analogs of the latest diabetes drugs without their potential for liver damage or weight gain.

Cassia Nomame , Hama-cha, Kita; nomame herba; Mimosoides tea
Botanical Name
Cassia nomame
Cassia nomame is native to China and originally produced in the south of the Changjiang river. An extract of this herb is showing up in many weight loss and diet formulations. The claim is that Cassia nomame is a natural lipase inhibitor, which means it disrupts the digestive enzyme process to block fat from getting into the bloodstream. It also is said to have diuretic and stimulating properties. The most prevalent sources of information I have been able to find concerning this

herb are those who have a financial interest in selling it. While it may well work, documentation is thin for the most part.

Castor Oil
Botanical Name
Ricinus communis
One of the most time honored home remedies for constipation, castor oil was the bane of childhood for those of us who were subjected to a daily dose of this rather vile tasting oil. But don't let that dissuade you from using castor oil externally, it is a wonderful analgesic oil when applied externally for all kinds of pain including: sore muscles and arthritis pain, bruising, lower back pain, and nerve damage. Castor oil packs are well suited to the slow relief of chronic pain and swelling. Castor oil forms a protective surface when used in cosmetic and skin care formulations that acts as a protective barrier for skin.

Cat's Claw , una de gato
Botanical Name
Uncaria tomentosa
The stem and root of cat's claw are harvested in Brazil, Peru, and other parts of the Amazon region, where it is known as una de gato. This woody vine clings to the tallest trees by it's thorns or "claws". The bark is traditionally used for inflammatory arthritis and intestinal complaints such as stomach ulcers. In Austria and Germany, cat's claw

preparations are prescription only medications.

Alkaloids found in the bark and roots of Cat's Claw have been documented to stimulate the immune system. Studies indicate at least six of these oxindole alkaloids can increase immune function by up to 50% in relatively small amounts. This has led to its use around the world as an adjunctive treatment for cancer and AIDS as well as other diseases which negatively impact the immune system.

Catnip , Catmint, Nep,Catnep

Botanical Name

Nepeta cataria

A harmless high for felines and beneficial for humans. Catnip leaves contain considerable quantities of vitamins C and E, both excellent antioxidants. The primary phytochemicals, nepetalactone isomers, are mild sedatives, somewhat like the active ingredients in valerian. Catnip is a gentle but potent sleep-inducer for humans that calms without affecting you the next day. It soothes the nervous system and can safely help get a restless child off to sleep, in fact catnip, along with chamomile, is one of the most often recommended herbs for use in children's complaints.

Catnip teas have long been used in traditional herbal medicine to quell digestive disturbances, and reducing the pain of menstrual cramps. A hot cup of catnip tea is excellent for treating colds and flu because it producing perspiration without increasing the heat of the system. Catnip tea is good for curing headaches as well.

Catuaba , caramuru, catagu, catigu, catigua, chuchuhuasha, pau de reposta, or tatuaba
Botanical Name
Erythroxylum catuaba
Syn. Trichilia catigua, Anemopaegma mirandum
Catuaba is the most famous of the Brazilian aphrodisiac plants, noted for it's ability to strengthen erections. Catuaba is an aphrodisiac that is useful in the treatment of impotence and prostatitis, and has been studied for possible benefits as a protective against opportunistic infection in HIV/AIDS. In 2002, a Brazilian company was awarded a patent for an HIV prevention formula based on an extract of the herb, although research is still in progress.

Cayenne Pepper , Capsicum ,African Pepper, Chillies, Bird Pepper
Botanical Name
Capsicum minimum
Heart Health: Cayenne is considered to be a valuable heart tonic. These hot peppers contain capsicum which has been shown to reduce cholesterol and triglyceride levels. Cayenne also helps to increase circulation and keeps the blood flowing smoothly through veins and arteries. Cayenne also is high in antioxidants, rounding out its cardiovascular benefits.
Hot, stimulating Cayenne peppers are like a jump start to a

cold car engine on a frosty morning. It brings welcome life into sore muscles and get your heart beating faster, increasing the flow of blood all through the body. The heat of cayenne warms stiff arthritic joints and relaxes away low back pain. The longer you use it, the better it works. Cayenne works very well for me, I use it every day, sometimes twice a day, for arthritis stiffness, sore muscles, and low back pain. Cayenne infused oil does not burn my skin as much as capsaicin creams. Cayenne salves and oils are my first recommendation to anyone who has problems with pain, however cayenne has many other varied uses that make it one of the most powerful remedies in your kitchen medicine cabinet.

Cayenne for Pain relief Cayenne pepper extracts are an important part of herbal treatment for muscle pain, fibromyalgia, arthritis, and the nerve pain caused by shingles and sciatica. It appears to act by decreasing the concentration of substance P, the primary chemical used by nerve cells to transmit pain signals. It takes repeated use over a period of at least a few weeks to feel this benefit. Cayenne is also rich in salicylates, natural aspirin like compounds, which add to its analgesic nature. Cayenne pepper balms, oils and creams are rubefacients, which means it warms the body by quickly dilating small capillaries, and increasing circulation, which reddens, (but does not burn) the skin. This increased circulation is the hallmark of cayenne's effect on the body, it stimulates the heart, and the lungs as well as increasing blood circulation and warmth throughout the whole system.

Cayenne Pepper Diet: Adding cayenne to your diet plan is a given. Cayenne, along with other peppers strengthen digestion and lessen the change of bacterial infections from unsanitary food and water. Cayenne peppers also lessen the gas and bloating that comes from eating heavy, greasy foods. Cayenne helps boost your metabolism and induces the body to burn off more fat. Eating more hot spicy foods will help decrease appetite and increase satiety, so you are inclined to eat less. Seasoning with pepper lessens the need for salt and fat in cooking without sacrificing flavor.

Psoriasis Treatment: Capsaicin, the most potent constituent of cayenne, has been shown to be effective in treating the symptoms of psoriasis. Treatment does produce burning sensations, which are normal and decrease with repeated use. If you buy OTC products look for one that contains menthol, it will help relieve the itching as well. A 1999 study found that treatment with capsaicin caused a marked decrease in psoriasis activity and decreased formation of new skin plaques.

Cedarwood, Atlas , Atlas cedar

Botanical Name

Cedrus atlantica

There are two commercial oils which are known as cedarwood today, Cedrus atlantica, Atlas cedarwood, which is a true cedarwood, and Juniperus virginiana, known as red cedar. Cedarwood is known for use in problem skin, as an insect repellent, and as an inhalant in respiratory complaints. It's actions are sedative, astringent, and antiseptic. It can be used to treat oily skin and scalp, relieve itching, and more serious skin conditions like psoriasis and eczema, remembering that high concentrations will irritate the skin. Cedarwood is similar in action to the highly expensive sandalwood, it also has a sedative effect making it grounding in conditions of anxiety and nervous tension.

Celandine , Greater or common celandine
Botanical Name
Chelidonium majus
Traditional Chinese medicine uses celandine in cough medicines, as the herb acts as an expectorant, and pain reliever.

Celery Seed
Botanical Name
Apium graveolens
Celery is a healthy medicinal food, often used to reduce the need for salt in cooking. The seeds contain apigenin and isoquerticin, compounds that help blood vessels to expand, lowering blood pressure. A natural diuretic, celery can reduce excess water buildup and decrease the uric acid that causes pain and inflammation in gout and arthritis.

Chaga Mushroom , Cinder conk, Birch mushroom
Botanical Name
Inonotus obliquus
Chaga was documented by Chinese herbalist Shen Nong in his herbal texts as early as the first century B.C.E. Russian folk medicine used chaga for ailments of the stomach, liver, and heart, as well as a tonic, blood purifier, and pain reliever. Chaga remains popular in Russia today, where it is sold as Befunigin, as a cancer cure.
Chaga mushrooms, or cinder conks, have been a staple of traditional medicine for centuries among the peoples of the boreal forests in Siberia, Asia and North America. They are used as a tonic and blood purifier. They belong to the Polypores, a group of mushrooms that grow on wood and may be the ancestors of most gilled mushrooms. Chaga and the similar reishi mushroom both have a reputation as tonics for longevity and health which are born out by recent scientific studies. These mushrooms show great promise for their anti-viral activities, immune response stimulation and anti-tumor effects that inhibit the spread of cancer cells.

Chamomile , Camomile, Chamomilla, German chamomile
Botanical Name
Matricaria recutita
Syn. M. chamomilla
Beautiful skin and hair: Chamomile contains compounds that are antibacterial and anti-inflammatory; one of these, the

lovely blue chamazulene, is noted for promoting tissue regeneration. The anti-inflammatory effect of the essential oil applied topically improves skin regeneration. Skin washes and baths with chamomile tea can calm skin inflammations, as well as bacterial skin diseases. The anti-inflammatory effect of the essential oil applied topically improves skin regeneration and a cold compress does wonders for puffy eyes. Cooled chamomile tea used as a hair rinse brings on the highlights in blonde or light colored hair. Add lemon juice to enhance the effect. Chamomile flower extracts are helpful in managing eczema .

Chanca Piedra , phyllanthus, quebra pedra, kidney stone tree
Botanical Name
Phyllanthus niruri
The name of chanca piedra in Portuguese, quebra pedra means "stone breaker." This traditional native medicine is used to treat kidney stones in both human and veterinary herbal medicine. It is a favorite natural treatment for kidney problems in guinea pigs and hamsters. The antispasmodic activity of alkaloids in Phyllanthus sellovianus explained the popular use of the plant for kidney and bladder stones.

Chaparral , hediondilla, Shegoi
Botanical Name
Larrea tridentata
Chaparral has potent and long-lasting anti-inflammatory and

analgesic effects in the treatment of rheumatoid arthritis. Chaparel is one of the medicinal plants of the Southwest,(along with osha Ligusticum porteri and jojoba Simmondsia chinensis) with a long history of medicinal use. Chaparral herb should only be used externally in baths, and the tincture can be used to make creams and lotions. Applied to the skin, chaparral can have a remarkable healing effect on the skin. It is useful for eczema, psoriasis, and as an excellent antiseptic dressing for cuts, sores and bruises.

Chaste Tree , Vitex, Chasteberry, Monk's Pepper
Botanical Name
Vitex agnus-castus
Vitex neither represses sexual passion, as the ancient Greeks who gave it the name Agnus casus (chaste), believed, nor does it act as a true aphrodisiac. Vitex is a normalizing herb for the female reproductive system, a regulator of the hormonal balance of estrogen and progesterone. 1 This normalizing of hormones is what makes the herb valuable in treating painful and irregular menses, PMS, menopause and infertility. For chronic problems, it is most effective when taken over a prolonged period of time.

Chicory root , Succory, Blue Sailors
Botanical Name
Cichorium intybus
The dark, rich flavor of chicory is best known as a southern substitute for coffee, but herbalists value chicory as a bitter digestive tonic. Drinking chicory on a regular basis helps to rid your system of excess water and uric acid buildup without depleting potassium and other minerals, helping to support the liver and the heart. This also makes chicory a good beverage for those with rheumatism and gout. In this respect it mirrors and complements the properties of dandelion, with which it is often combined.

Rehmannia root , Chinese Foxglove, Shu Di Huang
Botanical Name
Rehmannia glutinosa
Rehmannia root is a very commonly used herb in traditional Chinese medicine. Know as or Di-huang, (earth yellow), prepared rehmannia is used for loss of blood, yin deficiency, lower back pain with kidney deficiency from overwork (it replenishes the vital essence of the kidneys),lumbago, cough, hectic fever, diabetes, urinary incontinence, deafness, uterine bleeding, vertigo, tinnitus, and for regulating menstrual flow. Rehmannia has astringent properties that make it useful in stopping bleeding. It helps to protect and support the liver and adrenal glands and is often found in energy tonic formulas to used to combat chronic fatigue.

Chrysanthemum , Mums, Ju Hua, Chu Hua,Florist's Chrysanthemum

Botanical Name

Chrysanthemum morifolium, C. sinense

Syn. Dendranthema morifolium

In traditional Chinese medicine Ju-hua is used in Chinese medicine in prescriptions for colds with wind, and heat, headache, inflamed eyes, swelling and pain in the throat, vertigo, tinnitus, sores such as boils, and tightness of the chest with anxiety. Chrysanthemum flowers soaked in rice wine are a historical restorative drink. Chrysanthemum is combined with Japanese honeysuckle in the treatment of high blood pressure.

Cilantro , Chinese parsley, cilantro

Botanical Name

Coriandrum sativum

Cilantro (leaves)and Coriander (seeds) and are names for different parts of the same plant, Coriandrum sativum, a naturally healing food in both forms. Cilantro is an excellent culinary herb that adds flavor to foods and improved digestion. There are both scientific studies, and anecdotal evidence to support cilantro's reputation as a powerful digestive aide. The herb may also have a protective effect when cooked and eaten with fish and other foods that may be contaminated with heavy metals.

Peruvian Bark , Red Bark. Jesuits' Powder. Cinchona Bark
Botanical Name
Cinchona spp
Jesuit's Powder, also called Peruvian Bark, or Cinchona, is the historical remedy for all forms of malaria. The powdered bark of this South American Andes tree is the source of quinine, which became famous for the treatment of malaria, fever and pain in the 17th century. Its main active principle, quinine, is now chemically synthesized. The term quinine comes from the Peruvian ghina, or quina-quina. Another compound in chinchona, quinidine, is now a standard anti-arrhythmic medication. Quinine is the source of the bitter taste in tonic water. The mixed drink gin and tonic originated in British colonial India when the British population would mix their medicinal quinine tonic with gin to make it more palatable.

Cinnamon , Cassia Bark, Sweet cinnamon
Botanical Name
Cinnamomum zeylanicum, C. cassia
Cinnamon and Diabetes: Diabetes is a growing and grave concern that has many people searching for natural and safe ways to treat and prevent it. Some very interesting recent research suggests that cinnamon cassia (Cinnamomum aromaticum) is effective in improving blood glucose control in patients with type 2 diabetes.
Antibacterial Power of Cinnamon: The simple touch of cinnamon infuses warmth and energy throughout your body.

As part of tea blends, cinnamon improves the taste of less tasty herbs and adds powerful antibacterial power to cold and flu remedies. Cinnamon essential oil is a reliable remedy for athletes foot but should only be applied to the skin when diluted with a carrier oil.
Whole cinnamon, taken in tea or tincture form, is an effective treatment for yeast infections that are resistant to treatment. It is useful as a treatment for thrush, an oral yeast infection, as well as for the gum disease gingivitis.

Lemongrass , lemongrass
Botanical Name
Cymopogon citratus, C.flexuosus
Lemongrass is a well known medicinal herb in the east, as well as being widely used in Thai, Indonesian, Vietnamese, and Caribbean cooking. In Ayurvedic medicine a preparation of lemon grass with pepper has been used for relief of menstrual troubles and nausea. Lemon grass is a mild diuretic and a digestive stimulant that promotes digestion of fats.

Clary Sage , Clarysage
Botanical Name
Salvia sclarea
Clary sage has a special affinity with the female system in general and is recommended for women who are experiencing hot flashes, pain and tension associated with menopause, menstrual problems and PMS. Clary sage oil's contains

sclareol which has an estrogen-like structure, contributing to clary's effectiveness in returning balance to the female reproductive system. Clary sage oil's antispasmodic properties relieve pain and menstrual cramping in massage oil blends.

Cleavers , Clivers, Goose Grass, Catchweed, Sweet Woodruff
Botanical Name
Galium aparine
Herbalists have long regarded cleavers as a valuable lymphatic tonic and diuretic. The lymph system is the body's mechanism to wash tissues of toxins, passing them back into the bloodstream to be cleansed by the liver and kidneys. This cleansing action makes cleavers useful in treating conditions like psoriasis and arthritis, which benefit from purifying the blood. Cleavers is a reliable diuretic used to help clean gravel and urinary stones and to treat urinary infections. In cats, these actions make cleavers a safe long-term aid in the treatment of feline lower urinary tract disease, and the herb may also be useful for chronic low-grade kidney inflammation. In studies cleavers extract lowered blood pressure without slowing heart rate or having any health-threatening side effects.

Club Moss , Wolf's Claw
Botanical Name
Lycopodium clavatum,
Syn. Huperzia serrata
In traditional Chinese medicine An ingredient in the Traditional Chinese Medicine remedy Qian Ceng Ta, club moss has been used for centuries to treat fever and inflammation.

Coca, cocaine , cocaine
Botanical Name
Erythroxylum coca
Coca leaves have been used as a stimulant by the indigenous people of Peru, Bolivia, and northern Argentina for centuries; it also has religious and symbolic significance.
The Coca-Cola Company buys 115 tons of coca leaf from Peru and 105 tons from Bolivia per year, which it uses as an ingredient in its Coca-Cola formula (famously a trade secret). The cocaine itself does not end up in the drink nowadays, however, and is generally sold to the pharmaceutical industry where it is used for various surgical procedures.

Codonopsis , Dang Shen, tangshen, Bastard Ginseng, bonnet bellflowers
Botanical Name
Codonopsis pilosula
In traditional Chinese medicine As a cooling herb, codonopsis is useful in any illness in which "spleen qi deficiency" a

deficiency of digestive energies, is the underlying cause. Codonopsis is a relatively inexpensive herb that is often substituted for Panax ginseng in herbal tonics. It is believed to have an action similar to that of panax ginseng, but milder. Often used by poorer Chinese patients, it is commonly referred to as "poor man's ginseng". It's relatively low cost does not diminish it's place as one of the more important Chinese herbal medicines.

Coffee , java, joe
Botanical Name
Coffea arabica
The caffeine in coffee and tea is a chemical cousin to the asthma drug theophylline, drinking coffee and caffeinated teas can help calm an asthma attack and stop coughing spasms. Doctors at the Diamond Headache Clinic in Chicago, Illinois, have found that the common painkiller, ibuprofen, is more active against tension headaches when combined with caffeine.

Coleus Forskohlii , Forskolin, Indian Coleus, False Boldo
Botanical Name
Plectranthus barbatus
Coleus forskohlii has been traditionally used to treat high blood pressure. Other benefits include help in losing weight by improving the breakdown of fats, improving digestion and nutrient absorption, lowering cholesterol, and immune system

support. The active photochemical in Coleus forskohlii, forskolin, also helps people with asthma.

Comfrey Leaf and root
Botanical Name
Symphytum officinale
Syn. Symphytum uplandica x
Comfrey is a marvelous herb and is one of the best-known healing herbs of all times. Well known and widely used by early Greeks and Romans, its very name, symphytum , from the Greek symphyo means to "make grow together", referring to its traditional use of healing fractures. Comfrey relieves pain and inflammation caused by injuries and degeneration, especially the symptoms of rheumatoid arthritis and osteoarthritis. Comfrey creams and oils can be used in arthritic pain relieving massages. In a recent study patients with painful osteoarthritis of the knee treated with comfrey root extract in an ointment showed a reduction in pain , mobility of the knee improved and quality of life increased.

Coptis , Chinese goldthread, Huang Lian, Figwortflower,Canker Root
Botanical Name
Coptis spp
Coptis chinensis is used in traditional Chinese medicine, and is better known in Asia than in North America, that relies on native herbs like goldenseal.

It is used in much the same manner as other berberine containing herbs; barberry, goldenseal, and Oregon grape root. These herbs are used in treating and preventing infections and for supporting the immune system. The anti-inflammatory, antibiotic and anti-tumor effects of berberine are well documented, and Coptis chinensis, or Chinese goldthread, has been the subject of much cancer research in Japan and China.

Coriander , Chinese parsley, Cilantro
Botanical Name
Coriandrum sativum
The Coriandrum sativum plant produces both Coriander (seeds) and Cilantro (leaves) Coriander's anti-inflammatory properties can help reduce joint swelling in rheumatoid arthritis, a traditional use that has been recently validated in studies.

Corydalis , fumewort, Yan Hu So
Botanical Name
Corydalis spp
In traditional Chinese medicine Corydalis, yanhusuo, is used in traditional Chinese medicine as a pain reliever, and according to Chinese research, Corydalis has an analgesic effect approximately 1 % that of the strength of opium. Yuanhu Zhi Tong Formula, a combination of Angelica and Corydalis root is a traditional formula is in traditional Chinese medicine to soothe the Qi energy and prevent blood stagnation during pain.

Corydalis is a member of the poppy family, and like many Papaverceae Corydalis is an anodyne, a central nervous system depressant, cardiotonic, and sedative. Corydalis has been used and studied mostly in the East, and has been used in Chinese medicine for centuries. Corydalis is currently being studied for use in cancer, dysmenorrhea, hypertension, and convulsions, however the primary focus is on the herbs use as a natural pain reliever. It holds special promise for those with persistent, low-level chronic pain. This means it has the potential to offer relief of chronic, agonizing pain from arthritis to back pain.

Corydalis contains the alkaloid bulbocapnine, which is occasionally used in medicine to treat convulsions, Parkinson's disease and Meniere's disease. It has been used in the treatment of muscular tremors and vestibular nystagmus.

Damiana

Botanical Name

Turnera diffusa

Syn. Turnera diffusa Willd. ex Schult. var. aphrodisiaca

Damiana is used primarily as an aphrodisiac for both sexes , and as a stimulant that can boost mental focus and stamina. The health benefits of damiana are for the most part only verified by folklore and long observation, not by scientific study, however chemical analysis shows that damiana contains alkaloids similar to caffeine that have stimulating and aphrodisiac effects, stimulating blood flow to the genital area and increasing sensitivity. Some people report feelings of mild euphoria.

Dandelion Root , Priest's crown, Swine's Snout
Botanical Name
Taraxacum officinale
The Chinese dandelion, Chin Hung ,Taraxacum mongolicum, is used by them as a specific for appendicitis, and has been used to treat infections, particularly mastitis.
Acne and skin care Like burdock, dandelion root helps the body dispose of unwanted skin bacteria. It also stimulates digestion and supports the liver - the major organ that helps rid the body of toxins and excess hormones, including the androgens that trigger acne breakouts. As a specific herb for the liver, it also benefits the female reproductive system by helping to regulate and normalize hormone production.

Devil's Claw , grapple plant, wood spider
Botanical Name
Harpagophytum procumbens
Devils claw tubers contain a group of chemicals called iridoids that have anti-inflammatory activity, the two active ingredients in devil's claw are harpagoside and beta sitosterol. This herb has an extensive history of use as an anti-inflammatory, pain reliever, and digestive stimulant.
Devils claw offers slow but sure relief of joint pain caused by both osteoarthritis and rheumatoid arthritis, and it has also

been shown to relieve muscle pain and enhance mobility for people with either arthritis or muscle injuries. Scientists don't know exactly how devil's claw works at this time, other than that it is not a COX-2 inhibitor and therefore is not potentially injurious to the heart.

Because improper digestion of protein plays a role in gout, causing the uric acid buildup, this is a remedy tailor-made for people with gout.

Dong Quai , Chinese Angelica, Dang-gui

Botanical Name

Angelica sinensis

For over two thousand years, since the writing of the Divine Husband's Classic of the Materia Medica, Chinese herbal medicine has used dong quai to help women return to their natural hormonal and emotional states after the accumulation of toxins and emotional injuries in the energy organ known as the liver.

Elecampane , Wild sunflower, Horseheal, Yellow Starwort

Botanical Name

Inula helenium

In China, the native species of elecampane is called Hsuan-Fu-Hua. Chinese herbalists use elecampane root to treat pulmonary disorders, asthma and bronchitis.

Eleuthero Root , Siberian ginseng, Ci-wu-jia, Wu Jia Shen Jing
Botanical Name
Eleutherococcus senticosus
Syn. eleutherococcus
In traditional Chinese medicine Known in China as wu-jia-pi, eleuthero has been used in Chinese medicine for over 2,000 years, to balance vital energy and vitality. The herb is also commonly prescribed to treat respiratory and other infections. In traditional Chinese medicine, eleuthero is considered good for vital energy (qi/chi), used for sleeplessness with many dreams, lower back or kidney pain, deficiency of yang in the kidney or spleen, lack of appetite, and to enhance overall resistance to disease or stress. For treating rheumatoid arthritis and making muscles and bones strong, one prescription mixes wu-jia-pi with sweet rice wine.

Epimedium , horny goat weed, xian ling pi, and yin yang huo
Botanical Name
Epimedium grandiflorum
Traditional Chinese medicine practitioners use this herb used to increase the Yang energies, for instance, it would be used to enhance male sexual performance. Recent research has confirmed that Yin Yang Huo can increase sperm production and stimulate sexual desire.
Epimedium, also known as Yin Yang Huo or Horny Goat Weed, is a powerful remedy in traditional Chinese medicine and has been used for thousands of years to promote male potency,

libido, and as an aphrodisiac. Modern Chinese herbal medicine uses epimedium (usually in combination with other herbs) not just to treat impotence, but also for asthma, bronchitis, cervical dysphasia, congestive heart failure, leucorrhoea, leukopenia, and viral infections of the heart.

Epimedium is used to treat menopause in women often combined with Morinda. It is officially listed by the Chinese Academy of Medial Sciences as one of an elite group of herbs that slow down aging and promote longevity. Perhaps even more important have been the recent discoveries that Epimedium has powerful immune-modulating activity.

Evening Primrose Oil , Night Willow-herb

Botanical Name

Oenothera biennis

Borage is a member of the same family as comfrey. The plant contains potassium and calcium combined with mineral acids. Borage leaf may be useful for gently strengthening adrenal functions, the older herbalist wrote glowing accounts of the invigorating properties of the fresh leaf. "According to Dioscorides and Pliny, Borage was the famous Nepenthe of Homer, which when drunk steeped in wine, brought absolute forgetfulness."

Evening primrose seeds contain a fragrant oil that plays an important part natural health. The seed oil contains gamma-linolenic acid (GLA), an omega-6 fatty acid that the body uses to manufacture a prostaglandin vital to soothing inflammation and supporting the immune system. It also helps keep the blood flowing freely, reduces high blood pressure, plays a role in reducing breast cancers, and lowers cholesterol.

Fenugreek
Botanical Name
Trigonella foenum-graecum
Fenugreek is a medicinal food plant that has the beneficial effect of lowering blood sugar. The bitter seeds called methi in India, are used as a condiment and the leaves are used in teas. Fenugreek contains potent antioxidants that have beneficial effects on the liver and pancreas, making it useful in the treatment of diabetes, high cholesterol, and digestive disorders.

Feverfew
Botanical Name
Tanacetum parthenium
Feverfew inhibits platelet aggregating in the bloodstream, thus preventing blockage of small capillaries. This action is one of the reasons behind feverfew's popularity in treatment of migraines. It has a mild tranquilizing effect and is especially good for headaches caused by tension or fatigue. Feverfew has been used in the treatment of headaches since the first century. It has also been used for inflammation, arthritis, menstrual discomforts, fever, and other aches and pains.

Figwort , Carpenter's square

Botanical Name

Scrophularia nodosa

The name Scrophularia comes from scrofula, a form of tuberculosis that figwort was historically used to treat. Figwort is widespread in the Northern hemisphere, native species are found both in Europe, North America, (Scrophularia marilandica), and Asia that are very similar. Figwort was used to treat diseases of the throat. The herb was and is still used in salves and poultices to soothe inflamed skin in cases of psoriasis and eczema, and to heal burns. Herbalists today consider figwort as a cleansing herb that supports the detoxification of the body. Taken with salt it is a yin tonic.

Fo-Ti Root , Ho-shou-wu

Botanical Name

Polygonum multiflorum

Syn. Fallopia multiflora

The Chinese attributed mysterious anti-aging properties to the root of Polygonum multiflorum with the oldest (300 years) and biggest deemed "mountain spirit", mighty roots that literally bestowed immortality on the user. In Traditional Chinese Medicine fo-ti is one of the herbs used to nourish the heart and calm the spirit.

Fo-ti, as it is known here in the west is most famous for its reputed ability to restore color to gray hair and as a fertility tonic. It is prescribed in traditional Chinese medicine to unblock the channels of energy (meridians of ch'i) through the body, allowing the escape of the pathogenic influences that cause generalized weakness, soreness, pain, and fatigue.

Coleus Forskohlii , Forskolin, Indian Coleus, False Boldo
Botanical Name
Plectranthus barbatus
Coleus forskohlii has been traditionally used to treat high blood pressure. Other benefits include help in losing weight by improving the breakdown of fats, improving digestion and nutrient absorption, lowering cholesterol, and immune system.
Forsythia Fruit , Lian Qiao, yellow bell
Botanical Name
Forsythia suspensa
One of the 50 fundamental herbs in Chinese herbalism. The fruit of this olive relative is used to treat colds, viral infections, and fevers in traditional Chinese medicine.
Forsythia bushes are a popular ornamental here in the West, and like many other popular ornamental plants, forsythia has a long history of medicinal use in its Native China. Forsythia fruit is combined with another backyard favorite, honeysuckle, in one of the most widely used cold remedies in China.

Garlic , Poor Man's Treacle, Bawang, Bauang

Botanical Name

Allium sativum

Today garlic has found new respect from the modern scientific community for use in serious illness as well. Garlic contains allicin, a most impressive broad-spectrum antimicrobial as well as over thirty other medicinal compounds. Garlic and onions have long been used to treat bronchitis, allergies and asthma by helping to open the lungs and ease breathing. The ingredients responsible include mustard oils and quercetin. Garlic belongs to the allium genus which includes onions, shallots, leeks, scallions, and chives. This group of herbs are important in improving the digestibility of meats and other heavy foods and well as adding other healthy antioxidant and antimicrobial properties to your home cooking.

Garlic as a medicinal food has an impressive range of benefits. Garlic and its cousin onion contain substances that discourage platelets from sticking together and prevent blood clots, helping to naturally thin the blood. They also lower total cholesterol and triglycerides, another type of blood fat, all the while increasing HDL, "good cholesterol". Garlic may also lower blood-sugar levels in people with diabetes. Garlic may exert its effects in part by stimulating beta-cell insulin secretion. While garlic has had some mixed results in trials set to measure its effects on lowering blood sugar, diabetics may still wish to consciously add more fresh garlic to food, or even consider supplementation with garlic powder due to its protective health benefits and absence of major side effects. The major drawback to garlic continues to be the risk of stomach upset with higher doses, along with the usual risk of compounding the effects of prescription blood thinners.

Gentian , wild gentian ,yellow gentian

Botanical Name

Gentiana lute

In both Chinese and Korean, the terms for gentian can be translated literally as "dragon gallbladder herb." This attests to gentian's ability to treat fiery inflammations of the gallbladder that cause intense discomfort.

Gentian herb has been used in European and Eastern herbal medicine throughout the 3,000 years since its discovery to treat gallbladder problems and as a bitter tonic.

Ginger Root , Luyang Dilaw

Botanical Name

Zingiber officinale

The Chinese names for ginger Gan-jiang dried ginger, and Sheg-jiang, fresh ginger, mean to defend, suggesting that ginger helps protect the body from cold. Pulverized fresh ginger applied as a poultice to the head two to three times a day was once used as a (Chinese) folk treatment for baldness, and fresh ginger rubbed on the affected area is a folk remedy for vitiligo. The juice squeezed from the fresh root has also been used in the treatment of burns. In modern China ginger is probably used in half of all Chinese herbal prescriptions. Chinese healers believe than even moderate amounts of ginger tea strengthen the lungs and the kidneys.

Ginkgo biloba
Botanical Name
Ginkgo biloba L.
The earliest know reference to ginkgo is in the Chinese Materia Medica, in approx 2,800 B.C and the seeds and root have been used in traditional Chinese medicine for thousands of years to combat mental decline.
Ginkgo's hallmark effect is increased circulation, which is important in maintaining our energy level and one of the factors in stopping early hair loss. Increasing genital blood flow heightens responsiveness, making for higher libido in both men and women. Good circulation means getting the full benefit from the foods we eat and the vitamins and herbal supplements we take. Recently Ginkgo leaf has been studied for its cardiovascular benefits as well as brain function.

Ginseng root , Ren-shen, X-yang-shen, Asian ginseng, Korean ginseng
Botanical Name
Panax ginseng
Ginseng is a heat raising tonic for the blood and circulatory systems. Ginseng is one the best known and widely prescribed herbs in Chinese medicine as a general adaptogenic and

restorative tonic. Adaptogens such as ginseng are highly regarded in both Western and Eastern traditions for use in debilitated persons suffering from exhaustion, fatigue, liver disease, stress and wasting from chronic disease. Ginseng may boost mood and improve memory and attention spans for those under stress. Although the exact mechanisms of activity are not known, it is likely that ginseng protects a portion of the brain known as the hippocampus from the effects of stress hormones. Ginseng enhances the immune response which helps fight off viruses and bacteria. Ginseng is one of the best known herbal tonics used to restore libido in men without an increase in testosterone, which can aggravate prostate disorders. Unfortunately, the fame of ginseng has led to misconceptions about its use and to low grade or adulterated products being sold as ginseng in the West.

Panax, the generic name is derived from the Greek Panakos (a panacea), in reference to the miraculous virtue ascribed to it by the Chinese, who consider it a sovereign remedy in almost all diseases. The word Ginseng is said to mean wonder of the world, however, it is not universally applicable in every illness. It should not be taken during acute inflammatory disease or bronchitis since it can drive the disease deeper and make it worse. Chinese medicine considers ginseng to be one of the most yang herbs, suited to health problems related to a deficiency, or frailty (considered to be more yin). For someone with a very strong yang condition, the effects of ginseng will hardly be noticeable and is actually contraindicated for those whose yang condition is causing high blood pressure. This may explain the conflicting reports here in the West on whether ginseng is a cure for high blood pressure, or worsens it. Moreover, in China, ginseng is rarely used on its own, but is usually combined with other herbs, such as licorice or Chinese dates, which temper its powerful nature. Most herbalists recommend taking periodic rests from ginseng as it can raise anxiety levels in some people.

Eleuthero Root , Siberian ginseng, Ci-wu-jia, Wu Jia Shen Jing
Botanical Name
Eleutherococcus senticosus
Syn. eleutherococcus
Known in China as wu-jia-pi, eleuthero has been used in Chinese medicine for over 2,000 years, to balance vital energy and vitality. The herb is also commonly prescribed to treat respiratory and other infections. In traditional Chinese medicine, eleuthero is considered good for vital energy (qi or chi), used for sleeplessness with many dreams, lower back or kidney pain, deficiency of yang in the kidney or spleen, lack of appetite, and to enhance overall resistance to disease or stress. For treating rheumatoid arthritis and making muscles and bones strong, one prescription mixes wu-jia-pi with sweet rice wine.

Goji Berries , Lycii berry, Boxberry, Boxthorn, Wolfberry
Botanical Name
Lycium barbarum
Syn. Lycium chinense
A yin cooling tonic. Goji berries are valued in Chinese medicine and are used to strengthen the immune system, as a sexual tonic, improve vision, and as a liver and kidney tonic.
Goji are also called Chinese wolfberries and are an important part of Eastern cuisine.

Gotu Kola , Indian Pennywort, Brahmi
Botanical Name
Centella asiatica (L.)
Syn. Hydrocotyle asiatica
Gotu kola is an excellent vasodilator and blood vessel strengthener. The herb is also often used as a diuretic, antioxidant, and anti-inflammatory. This herb facilitates the actions of the antioxidant vitamins C and E in areas where there is damage. Gotu kola is widely used in Ayurvedic medicine and traditional Chinese medicine to rejuvenate both mind and body, and can be used in conjunction with bacopa, or Brahmi, another Ayurvedic herb used to improve mental focus and improve memory. Clinical experiments have shown that the plant rejuvenates skin and body tissue by stimulating collagen synthesis. Gotu kola's constituents of primary pharmacological interest are its “triterpenoids”, which have been shown to exert a complex set of actions on cells and

tissues, particularly connective tissues, participating in the healing process.
This herb was used by the legendary Li Ching-Yuen who died May 6, 1933, was a Chinese herbalist who supposedly lived to be over 256 years old! He claimed to be born in 1736, while disputed records suggest 1677.*

*Learn more about Li Ching-Yuen, and more about longevity on the "Longevity and legends" chapter.

Tea , Green Tea, Black tea
Botanical Name
Camellia sinensis
Chinese legend dates green tea back to 2737 BC. Green tea is currently being studied for its beneficial uses, and as a treatment for a number of different conditions and illnesses. Most of the western world drinks black tea while much of Asia, the Middle East and northern Africa drinks green tea. All teas come from the same plant, Camellia sinensis, the different coloring is due to different processing of the teas. The current "weight loss" use may be due to the fact that people are drinking more green tea, and less or no more soda's.

Gurmar
Botanical Name
Gymnema sylvestre
Gurmar (Gymnema sylvestre) has a long history of use in Ayurvedic medicine for the treatment of diabetes, upper respiratory infections, and fevers. The main point of interest in the west is gurmar leaf's effects on insulin levels and blood sugar given the rising epidemic of adult onset type 2 diabetes. Gurmar acts to normalize blood sugar levels only lowering glucose in those who are hyperglycemic. This herb also has a positive effect on triglycerides and cholesterol levels as well. Gurmar is of interest to dieters as well. Taken over a long period of time it has been shown to reduce the sugar cravings that can hijack your sensible eating plans.

Jiaogulan , Jiao Gu Lan, Amachazuru, Herb of Immortality, sweet tea vine
Botanical Name
Gynostemma pentaphyllum
The Chinese named the plant xiancao, "herb of immortality", due to the long life spans of those in Southern China who consumed it. Jiaogulan received only passing mentions in the classical Chinese medical texts, that were written mainly from the perspective of central and northern China.
Jiaogulan is a member of the cucumber family that is native to Asia, and has been used as a medicinal folk tea in Southern China for many years. Research (mostly from China and

Japan), has confirmed some of the therapeutic qualities of jiaogulan tea. Jiaogulan (Jiao Gu Lan)is an adaptogen and antioxidant whose chemical constituents (saponins) have properties similar to that of ginseng. The herb tea is valued for it's antioxidant protection, cardiovascular benefits. It reduces the negative effects of stress, has a normalizing effect on blood pressure, and thins the blood. Daily use of the tea may even help increase the metabolism of fats, and be used in successful weight loss programs. Daily use of the tea may not guarantee an immortal life-span, but this tasty brew is great for your heart.

Hemp Oil
Botanical Name
Cannabis sativa
Syn. C.sativa ssp. indica
Hemp, (Cannabis sativa), seed is a highly nutritious food, and contains anti-oxidants, protein, carotene, phytosterols, phospholipids, as well as a number of minerals including calcium, magnesium, sulfur, potassium, iron, zinc, and phosphorus. It is a source of complete protein and contains all twenty know amino acids, including the nine essential amino acids. It also contains Vitamins A, B1, B2, B3, B6, C, D, and E. The green color in hemp seed oil is a result of the high level of chlorophyll which is naturally present in the seeds. Hemp seed oil is a luxurious skin treatment and may suppress convulsions in children and young adults.

Perhaps the most valued property of (Cannabis sativa) is its percentage of essential fatty acids, which is higher than any other plant in the world. It contains both Omega-6 and Omega-3 Essential Fatty Acids, in a proportion of 3:1. This proportion is the recommended balance of Omega-6 to Omega-3 acids, making it a simple perfect way to complete your diet. Essential fatty acids are necessary for our health, and are responsible for the luster in our skin, hair, eyes, transferring oxygen to the every cell in our body, and even the clarity in our thought processes. Hemp seeds are comparable to sunflower seeds, and may be used for food and milk, tea, and for baking, like sesame seeds.

Hops , Hops
Botanical Name
Humulus Lupulus
Hops contains the most potent of all the plant estrogens, prenylnaringenin. For this reason, children of either sex who have not reached puberty should not be given hops. Limit use to small quantities of high quality formulations, or use fresh or dried hops with moderation.
Aged hops are sedatives, fresh hops provide bitters that stimulate digestion; these bitters are also found in the aged herb. In folk medicine, Hops teas are also used to relieve the pain of bladder infections and give prompt ease to an irritable bladder. Hops are a traditional cure for insomnia - a number of phytochemicals in hops are tonic, nervine and possess

sedative and muscle-relaxing qualities. Hops contain compounds that depress the central nervous system supporting its main use as a sedative. Hops can be combined with other herbs in anti-anxiety formulas that can be beneficial for sleeplessness and nervousness.

Ivy gourd
Botanical Name
Coccinia grandis
Ivy gourd is used in Ayurvedic medicine and Asian cuisine in a very similar manner to that of bitter melon. This very adaptable plant has been introduced to Hawaii as a food crop where it has become an invasive species. The plant has a potential hypoglycemic action in patients with mild diabetes.
Jamaican Dogwood , Florida Fishposion Tree
Botanical Name
Piscidia piscipula
Syn. P. erythrina
Jamaican dogwood is a fairly potent sedative well known as a specific for migraine headaches, neuralgia, and for treatment of insomnia caused by pain , nervous tension, and stress. The bark is anti-inflamatory and antispasmodic and can be used in cases of dysmenorrhea (painful periods). Jamaican dogwood is a strong analgesic that can be used along with other herbs to treat the musculoskeletal pain of arthritis and rheumatism.

Jasmine Flower Oil
Botanical Name
Jasminum officinale
For centuries in Egypt, India and the Orient, only the privileged upper classes were permitted access to the precious oil known as an aphrodisiac.
Legendary jasmine is a sensual delight, and is one of the principle oils used in perfumes and ointments for dry sensitive skin. In aromatherapy, jasmine absolute oil in used to uplift the spirits in cases of apathy, depression, menopausal disorders, and lack of confidence. A legendary aphrodisiac, jasmine's sweet scent has a profound effect on frigidity and impotence. It can relax the mother and help relieve the pain of childbirth and is thought to increase breast-milk.

Kava-Kava , Ava. Intoxicating Peper
Botanical Name
Piper methysticum
The word kava is used to refer both to the plant and the beverage produced from its roots. Kava kava can be used as a mild sedative for nervous tension and stress. The active constituents in the roots, kava lactones, have relaxing and intoxicating properties. Kava can be used as a relaxing, evening drink with friends, as long as it is used in a responsible manner.

Kudzu

Botanical Name

Pueraria lobata

In traditional Chinese medicine, where it is known as gat-gun,ge gan, kudzu is considered one of the 50 fundamental herbs. Traditional Chinese medicine uses kudzu in treating the symptoms of high blood pressure such as headache and dizziness (although kudzu has little or no effect on blood pressure itself). Kudzu powder is also taken internally on a regular basis to prevent recurrences of colds sores, shingles, and genital herpes.

Licorice Root , Liquorice, Gan-cao

Botanical Name

Glycyrrhiza glabr

In traditional Chinese medicine Gan-cao (licorice) is used in prescriptions for weak spleen and stomach energy, for coughs, sore throats, asthma, carbuncles, swelling with pain, sores with toxic matter, stomach ulcers, hepatitis, hysteria, and as a detoxicant for food or medicine poisoning, as well as to "mediate" or "harmonize" the poisonous character of toxic medicinal plants.

Maca root , Maca, Peruvian ginseng, maka
Botanical Name
Lepidium peruvianum
Syn. L weddellii, L. affine, L. gelidium
Maca has been growing in world popularity over the last several years due to its energizing and hormonal balancing properties. As a female tonic, maca may help with menstrual irregularities, female hormonal imbalances, and unwanted symptoms of menopause. Maca root is often combined with other herbs like Tribulus to help increase libido, and to assist both sexes in promoting a healthy sexual response.

Maitake mushroom , Hen of the Woods
Botanical Name
Grifola frondosa
Traditional Eastern medicine values maitake as an adaptogen, an aid to balance out altered body systems to a normal level, especially the immune system.

Muira puama , Marapama, potency wood
Botanical Name
Ptychopetalum olacoides
Folklore throughout South America strongly supports muira puama's stimulating properties. It is commonly referred to not only as an aphrodisiac but also as a nerve stimulant that is said to heighten the receptiveness to sexual stimuli, and muira puama is a preventive of baldness. Traditional healers

use all parts of the tree for food and medicine, but focus primarily on the bark and roots to make a tea taken to treat rheumatism, strengthen the heart, and promote intestinal health. It has been widely used in Europe and South America for hundreds of years and was listed in the British Herbal Pharmacopoeia as a treatment for impotence.

Oolong Tea , Wu Long, Wu Yi Tea
Botanical Name
Camellia sinensis
Oolong tea was first produced in the Wuyi Mountains at the beginning of the Qing Dynasty. Oolong (also spelt Wulong, or Wu Long) is literally 'black dragon' tea, but they say the name originally had nothing to do with dragons; rather, it was named after its discoverer Wu Liang.
Oolong tea is unique because of its partial fermentation which produces a diverse arrangement of both off-green and black leaves. This tea is beautiful, tasty, full bodied, healthy and with a mildly smooth aftertaste. The tea has become more popular in the West, marketed mainly as a diet aid, but just like green tea and all the different varieties of Camellia sinensis, oolong tea is rich in antioxidants that can help prevent cancer and heart disease and contribute to well-being. The health benefits add an extra layer of goodness to the simple enjoyment of the unique full bodied taste of oolong teas.

Passion Flower
Botanical Name
Passiflora incarnata
Herbalists have a high regard for the soothing properties of passionflower and recommend it as a general nerve tonic to treat nervous stress. Passionflower is used to gently relax the mind and body to prepare for a more restful nights sleep.

Pau d'arco , lapacho, taheebo
Botanical Name
Tabebuia spp
The Mayans and Incas of South America regarded Pau d'arco as an important healing herb, but the scientific study is still very preliminary; the bottom line is that pau d'arco seems to be more promising for fungal infections than malignant cancers. There is a great deal of practical evidence, however, that Pau d'arco can be used with success to treat colds, flu, sore throat, and yeast infections. Laboratory evidence suggests that the herb contains compounds that protect against tropical diseases, specifically malaria, schistosomiasis, and tropical fevers. The herb is added to ointments to treat psoriasis, and taken orally to relieve ulcers.

Pygeum
Botanical Name
Prunus africanum
Syn. P. africana
The terpenes in pygeum have an anti-swelling effect. Terpenes are present in many plants that produce fragrant essential oils. Prostaglandins are inflammatory hormones that tend to accumulate in the prostates of men with BPH. Research indicates that the phytosterols in pygeum interfere with the formation of these prostaglandins, helping to reduce inflammation and swelling of the prostate. When taken correctly, pygeum is considered one of the safest herbs used for male health, and often is combined with saw palmetto.

Reishi Mushroom , Ling-zhi, ling chih, ling chi mushroom
Botanical Name
Ganoderma lucidum
Cordyceps is another immune-modulating medicinal mushroom that possesses anti-tumor properties and stimulates tumor necrosis factor, a cytokine protein that destroys cancer cells. The name cordyceps in Chinese literally means "winter bug summer herb." It is an antlered fungus that grows in insect larvae, usually before the insect's cocoon is formed. Cordyceps relieves conditions that traditional Chinese medicine associates with the kidneys, including high cholesterol and ringing in the ears. The herb is an aphrodisiac that has been used as a cure for impotence.

Reishi, or Ling zhi is the extract of the Ganoderma lucium mushroom. This mushroom has been used in traditional Chinese and Japanese medicines for thousands of years, who place it in the highest class of tonic medicines, those who benefit the vital life energy or Qi. Reishi mushrooms are commonly prescribed for a host of conditions such as anxiety, high blood pressure, bronchitis, insomnia, and asthma but is particularly renowned for its use in hepatitis and other diseases of the liver and for promoting longevity. Reishi is used to prevent "fatty-liver" and cirrhosis due to alcohol abuse.
The Western focus on reishi is on the mushroom's immuno-enhancing and anti-tumor activities, the exact mechanism is still unknown, but it is thought that the mycopolysaccharides contained in the cell walls may hold the key to the mushrooms medicinal properties.

Sage
Botanical Name
Salvia officinalis
The Chinese have long valued sage for its healing properties. Red sage or dan-shen Salvia miltiorrhiza is one of many Chinese species in the genus, and is a very commonly used in traditional Chinese herbal medicine to relieve pain after childbirth and regulate menstruation. Combined with dan-gui, it is used to regulate suppressed menstrual flow.
The Chinese believe that sage was the key to a long life. This is the same sage that in most modern kitchens rarley use. The

uses of sage outside of the kitchen range from the mundane to the mystical, from a cure for the common cold to the psychoactive effects of Salvia divinorum and Salvia apiana in ceremonial and religious celebrations.

Schisandra , Magnolia vine, wu-wei-zi, Schizandra
Botanical Name
Schisandra chinensis
Schisandra fruit is widely used as a male tonic and adaptogenic in China. The Chinese name, wu-wei-zi, means five taste fruits. Schisandra has an usually sour, sweet, bitter, warm, and salty taste, as such the herb considered balanced in traditional Chinese medicine by virtue of this distribution of flavors.

Schisandra is a well known in Chinese medicine as one of the adaptogenic herbs that help to improve mental function, reduce tiredness and improve endurance. Use the berries as a tea, extracts, or supplement with schisandra capsules as a long term tonic for chronic fatigue. Schisandra is also a well recognized lung tonic and is used in cough syrups and to help improve breathing.

Schisandra fruit is widely used as a male tonic and adaptogenic in China. The Chinese name, wu-wei-zi, means five taste fruits. Schisandra has an usually sour, sweet, bitter, warm, and salty taste, as such the herb considered balanced in traditional Chinese medicine by virtue of this distribution of flavors.

Schisandra is believed to have an adaptogenic function to increase non-resistant immune response, and may help enhance vision. Alcohol extracts of Schisandra have helped to regenerate liver tissue, and thus have been used clinically in China for infectious hepatitis.

Sesame
Botanical Name
Sesamum indicum
Sesame seeds and sesame seed oil are used for food and skin care and have a rich tradition of medicinal use. Sesame seeds are used in Chinese medicine as a treatment for hair loss, and as a liver tonic. Both ginger root and sesame are invigorating to the scalp and can stimulate hair growth. For a ginger oil treatment, grate fresh ginger root and mix it with sesame oil. Massage the ginger oil into your scalp and leave it on for about 10 minutes. Rinse and shampoo your hair.

Solomon's Seal
Botanical Name
Polygonatum biflorum
The leaves of Polygonatum resemble bamboo leaves, and the plant is known in the Chinese language as "jade bamboo,". It is a common plant in the mountains of northern China. The Chinese use the root of several polygonatum species as a cooling, demulcent, sedative, anti-periodic (preventing the periodic return of attacks of disease, as of certain fevers, esp.

malaria) and tonic. It was used to treat lung complaints, influenza, rheumatism and many other conditions.

Tribulus terrestris L , Burra Gookeroo, Burra Gokhru, puncture vine,

Botanical Name

Tribulus terrestris,

Syn. Pedalium Murex L

Tribulus relaxes smooth muscles and improves the circulation in the genital region of both men and women, leading to improved sexual response. For women, the hormone balancing effects of Tribulus terrestris make this a suitable herb for premenstrual syndrome and menopausal symptoms. Tribulus is also a popular anabolic supplement among body builders who use it to lower cholesterol and increase lean muscle mass.

Tribulus terrestris has anti-bacterial and anti-viral properties that may be used to treat herpes, and virus infections such as influenza and the common cold.

Yohimbe , johimbe, yumbina

Botanical Name

Pausinystalia johimbe

While Yohimbe herb is often thought of for male erectile dysfunction support, most people don't realize that yohimbe is also effective in women. This herb increases blood flow to the genitals of both males and females giving women an enhanced sensation and engorgement of genital organs. However, keep the dose low to prevent the yohimbe side effects. This effect lasts 2-3 hours before diminishing.

Yohimbe is also sold as a muscle building natural version of anabolic steroids. However, it's action is apparently unrelated to the body's production of testosterone, which means it probably is of little value in building bigger muscles.

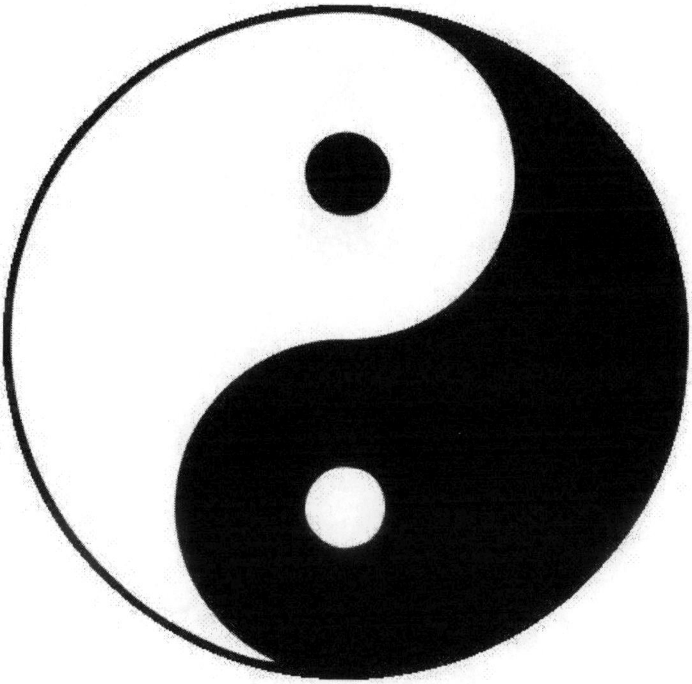

29448199R00104

Made in the USA
Charleston, SC
13 May 2014